Clinical Interviewing
and Counseling
PRINCIPLES AND TECHNIQUES

APPLETON PSYCHIATRY SERIES

Edited by

Thomas F. Dwyer, M.D.
Fred H. Frankel, M.D.

Department of Psychiatry,
Harvard Medical School,
Boston, Massachusetts

Clinical Interviewing and Counseling
PRINCIPLES AND TECHNIQUES

GOLDA M. EDINBURG, M.S.S.S., ACSW

Adjunct Assistant Professor, Boston University; Associate in Psychiatric Social Work, Simmons College, Boston, Massachusetts; Director, Social Work Department, McLean Hospital, Belmont, Massachusetts

NORMAN E. ZINBERG, M.D.

Associate Clinical Professor of Psychiatry, Harvard Medical School; Faculty, Boston Psychoanalytic Institute; Psychiatrist-in-Chief, Washingtonian Center for Addictions, Boston, Massachusetts; Senior Staff Psychiatrist, Department of Psychiatry, The Cambridge Hospital, Cambridge, Massachusetts

WENDY KELMAN, M.S.S.S., ACSW

Clinical Social Worker, Social Work Department, McLean Hospital, Belmont, Massachusetts

APPLETON-CENTURY-CROFTS/New York
A Publishing Division of Prentice-Hall, Inc.

Library of Congress Cataloging in Publication Data

Edinburg, Golda M
    Clinical interviewing and counseling.

    (Appleton psychiatry series)
    Includes bibliographies and index.
    1. Counseling. 2. Interviewing.   I. Zinberg, Nor-
man Earl, 1921-   joint author. II.   Kelman, Wendy,
1946-   joint author. III. Title.   [DNLM: 1. Counseling. 2. Interview, Psychological.   BF637.I5 E23c]
BF637.C6E34 1975   616.8'9'075   74-23099
ISBN 0-8385-1139-2

75 76 77 78 79/10 9 8 7 6 5 4 3 2

Acknowledgments

A book on clinical procedures requires the cooperation of many people. Our clients, our supervisors, our students, and our colleagues have contributed some of the actual incidents and techniques described here, but more than that they are responsible for our capacity to think through and understand technical responses and the theories that lead to those responses. Counselors, to practice comfortably, need a psychological aptitude; that is, an ability to think abstractly and sensitively about intrapsychic and interpsychic interactions. But given a bit of that capacity, counselors are made. They are made by their own interest and dedication and by the interest and dedication of their supervisors, clients, and colleagues. Hence, this book owes its principal debt to all the people who have worked in those capacities with the three of us over the years.

Other colleagues have contributed more specifically to the book itself. Professor Louise Frey, Director of Continuing Education at Boston University School of Social Work, reviewed Chapter 10, "Getting the Most out of Supervision," and her formulations of the problems involved in interviewing and counseling are present in other parts of the book. The sound advice and editorial comments of Dr. Thomas Dwyer, Director of the Psychiatric Training Program for Medical House Officers at Massachusetts General Hospital, have been used throughout the book to the extent that the tightness and consistency achieved are due to his attention. We are especially grateful to Mr. Donald Riley, Director of Staff Development of the Family Service Association of Greater Boston, for the confidence expressed in us by that agency's willingness to share case material.

Much appreciation is due to Ms. Edinburg's secretaries for their forbearance. Special thanks go to Ms. Helen Estey and Ms. Elizabeth Stein, who patiently typed and retyped these chapters to achieve readability.

Getting the ideas together in readable form has been a valuable experience for us. May it be so for the readers as well.

G. M. E.
N. E. Z.
W. K.

Contents

Introduction

The purpose of this book is to make explicit to beginning interviewers techniques that are often taken for granted by experienced therapists. The concept of translating "how to interview" into comprehensible language is the outgrowth of a seminar for social work students at McLean Hospital, in Belmont, Massachusetts, conducted by Golda M. Edinburg, Director of the Social Work Department.

The students in the seminar were unusually bright and well versed in theory. However, they seemed quite unaware of many of the practical approaches to and details of interviewing. It became obvious to Ms. Edinburg that many principles and techniques that she regarded as common sense and thus took for granted actually were grounded in a body of practical experience not yet a part of the beginner's skills. With his excessive concern and anxiety, the trainee has not yet integrated this body of skills. As a result, the relationship between the counselor and the client is often ambiguous and inconsistent.

The students were concerned about being able to maintain a useful relationship with a client. They were worried that the client, no matter how distressed, would know of their inexperience and disdain them. Therefore, they found it particularly difficult to confront clients with certain realities. For example, one student allowed his client to refer to him as doctor. He was afraid that if he clarified his status the client would automatically terminate the relationship. He had overlooked the fundamental principle that with so much ambiguity inherent in the therapeutic situation, it is important to clarify reality factors whenever possible. But when there is as much anxiety and uncertainty about what to do and when and how to do it as this student experienced, any basic principle can get lost.

The students in this seminar were not only troubled by status issues. Sometimes they refrained from asking obvious questions out of embarrassment and fear of being exposed as ignorant. Since it is essential for counselors to find out what they do not know, the principle of asking questions must be stressed to them.

As Ms. Edinburg became aware that basic principles such as asking questions and clarifying reality factors were not generally taught, she recognized the need for a handbook on clinical interviewing and counseling: a text that would provide beginners with an outline, rough and imprecise at best, but that would offer suggestions about what to do and when and how to do it. After completing her two-year placement, Wendy Kelman, one of the seminar students, joined the social work staff at McLean Hospital and began to work with Ms. Edinburg on the "guideline" project. They were joined in their endeavor by Dr. Norman Zinberg, a psychiatrist with many years of experience in teaching and supervising interviewing and counseling for a wide variety of professional and nonprofessional workers. Our aim was to provide a handbook that was not limited to a specific professional group. Many workers from different backgrounds are now employed by schools, hospitals, clinics, community agencies, rehabilitation services, and the like, who need an orientation to interviewing and counseling as much as the seminar students.

We began the project by reviewing the literature. The social work literature centered mainly on the helping process; that is , the worker is presented as being in a position to offer "help" to someone in need. Unfortunately the wish to "help" places a heavy responsibility on the beginner, who all too often takes on the "burden" of his client's problem. This can be infantilizing and patronizing to the "helpee," who is placed in a weak position. Instead of stressing the "helping relationship," we describe the "working relationship" (Chap. 3), which focuses on the alliance between two partners with equal but different tasks.

The extensive psychiatric literature was more theoretical and, hence, more difficult to translate into what, how, and when. It was more specifically aimed at residents in psychiatry or considerably more advanced therapists.

Clinical psychologists interestingly enough chose their major interviewing books from those written by psychiatrists rather than other psychologists. Nurses consistently referred to books written by nurses but also included material from the social work literature.

The books listed in the Bibliography following the Introduction, as well as this handbook, are limited to a consideration of the one-to-one relationship. Even though the counselor most frequently works with an individual client, the client needs to be considered within the context of his family, his culture, and his society or environment. There may be times when it is desirable for the counselor to see the entire family in the office or in the client's home to assess a situation or discuss a recommendation. Interviewing an entire family no matter where it takes place presents a special challenge to the beginner. Not only must he take into account the various dynamics of the individuals involved, but he must also consider the complications of the group or family process. We will not discuss family treatment per se. However, we consider the individual as a member of a family or a group; that is, his social reality is always taken into account.

Although the interest in preparing this book was stimulated by a social work seminar, the decision to actually complete the work came from another social reality. The mental health field was and is clearly changing. There is a burgeoning group of mental health workers who do not have a specific professional background or direct access to seminars or courses. In reviewing the literature, we were convinced that with only a few exceptions the texts were expected to be accompanied by a more formal curriculum. We believe that the theoretical and practical base for interviewing need not be presented in so abstract a form. But we also believe that without some source of instruction in technique, the zeal and good intentions of these beginning workers will not be enough. It is not a new problem. Social workers in the 1920's faced the same situation when they turned to a psychoanalytic dynamic model for help in understanding the irrational unconscious forces that impeded the client's progress.* This conceptual model, with all its intricacies, is inherently a complex one. At that time, books and courses had to be specially designed for the new entrants into the field, just as now we must prepare to train and educate another wave of interviewers and counselors.

In this handbook we aim to present the complex relationship between conscious and unconscious forces so that it can be understood and used by colleagues entering clinical practice with or without a concurrent professional sequence. Throughout the book the existence of unconscious forces in both counselor and client is recognized and taken into account, but the descriptions stress the conscious interactions between them. Thus, the counselor will have examples of what he can do with a fair degree of confidence during his first few months of training even if he is on his own. If he has courses or seminars available to him, these examples can serve as takeoff points for discussion.

Without such understandable examples and some supervision, beginners often unwittingly depend on facets of their own personality to structure the interview. This personal intrusion may take the form of moralizing or

*Borenzweig H: Social work and psychoanalytic theory: a historical analysis. J Soc Work 16(1):7-9, January 1971

changing the subject as cues come from within the counselor rather than from the client. As a counselor obtains instruction and experience, his confidence in his ability to interview grows, and he is better able to differentiate his own feelings from those of the client. With this growing self-awareness, the counselor is able to better understand and make sense of what the client brings to the situation. We describe many typical situations and kinds of clients so that an interviewer, who is beginning to recognize what particular, and often repetitious, instances of client-counselor interactions are like, will have a framework on which to build his experience.

Fortunately, most beginners bring to the interview an intuitive grasp of what is going on. Their enthusiasm and genuine interest in the client, plus the ongoing opportunity for supervision, education, and practical training, usually compensate for their lack of skill. All of us in the field—counselors and clients—take comfort (but not, we trust, license) in the human capacity for resilience and the ability of clients to tolerate technical "mistakes" on the part of counselors and particularly new counselors. The slow development of competence and its accompanying professional sense of unity can be interfered with by perfectionist standards.

Because individuals are so splendidly different, our guidelines cannot cover every anticipated situation. Medical practice, agency rules, regulations, preferences, and limitations affect the counselor's services. In addition, supervision and training are necessary for the beginner, and the supervisor's views are another influence on the counselor's techniques. In the last analysis, it is necessary to use judgment, sensitivity, and intelligence in developing the capacity to understand what the client is implying, experiencing, and saying.

BIBLIOGRAPHY

not Behavioral Science,

Social Work Literature

Garrett A: Interviewing: Its Principles and Methods, 2nd ed. New York, Family Service Association of America, 1972

Hollis F: Casework: A Psychosocial Therapy. New York, Random House, 1969

Kadushin A: The Social Work Interview. New York, Columbia Univ Press, 1972

Reid WJ, Epstein L: Task-Centered Casework. New York, Columbia Univ Press, 1972

Schubert M: Interviewing in Social Work Practice: An Introduction. New York, Council on Social Work Education, 1971

Psychiatric Literature

Colby KM: A Primer for Psychotherapists. New York, Roland Press, 1951
Gill M, Newman R, Redlich F: The Initial Interview in Psychiatric Practice. New York, International Univ Press, 1954
MacKinnon RA, Michels R: The Psychiatric Interview in Clinical Practice. Philadelphia, Saunders, 1971
Sullivan HS: The Psychiatric Interview. New York, Norton, 1954
Whitehorn JC: Guide to interviewing and clinical personality study. Arch Neurol and Psychiatry 52:197-216, 1944

Nursing Literature

Bermosk L, Mordan, MJ: Interviewing in Nursing. New York, Macmillan, 1964
Peplau HE: Interpersonal Relations in Nursing. New York, Putnam's, 1952

Clinical Interviewing and Counseling
PRINCIPLES AND TECHNIQUES

1
THE THERAPEUTIC PROCESS

The base of any therapeutic interaction is the interview. The scope of this book will be limited to the one-to-one interview. As we view the therapeutic context, the roles of the client and counselor in the interviewing and counseling situation are clearly defined. The client seeks out the counselor and makes an appointment, thus explicitly or implicitly announcing that he has an emotional conflict to discuss.

It is usually after the client has made this essential step and has begun to talk that he is in for a surprise. Many clients come in expecting to be "worked on" by the counselor, rather than to *share* a period of work and discovery. Deep down most clients hope that they will be told what they do not know and what they *should* or *should not* think or do.

Most clients believe that the counselor will have words of wisdom and specific solutions for their problems. This is true even of sophisticated individuals who have had wide exposure to theories of treatment through books and through reports of their friends' experiences. The person who is hurt or troubled, anxious or depressed, wants a prescription that will take away the pain. Whereas the counselor knows beforehand that he has no special answers, the client is disappointed when the counselor offers few, if any, suggestions as to what the client should do to solve his problem. And it takes time in the treatment for the client to recognize that his hopes to be "cured" are themselves items to be worked on.

The client brings to the situation a variety of expectations, some of which are fulfillable and some of which are unfulfillable through the counseling process. Our technical suggestions are intended to provide the means with which to work with these unfulfillable expectations, not to fulfill them or decry them. The counselor has to keep a careful watch over what he explicitly or implicitly promises the client. He must not operate as a controlling, parental figure and decide what is "better" for a client. Instead, the counselor should help the client to understand more fully what goes into, or what inhibits, his finding or meeting his own life standards. In effect, the client learns about the process of making life decisions. But which decisions he makes are his own responsibility, as the counseling techniques make abundantly clear. Only the client can decide what is truly better for him.

Often a client finds it hard to share or to state clearly his conflicts. It may be difficult for him to differentiate between an internal conflict and a complicated external situation. Thus, it is important for the counselor to recognize when the main difficulty is not emotional confusion but instead confusion about knowing whom to contact for help with an external difficulty. The counselor is able to perform a specific task by referring the client to the appropriate agency when indicated. For example, a client may be wondering if she is pregnant and, if so, where to go. The counselor can discuss the client's concerns about being pregnant as part of a therapeutic interaction. He can also refer the client to a gynecological service for a medical examination.

Some clients make impossible demands. Their own emotional involvement in the problem makes them temporarily unable to think clearly.

> The father of a 16-year-old girl told the counselor that the only help he wanted was to get his daughter to move back home. The man's marital relationship was deteriorating because his wife was depressed and barely functioning due to continued worry about the girl. He felt that the girl's return was critical to saving his marriage. It was obvious to the counselor that he could not fulfill this client's demands. He could, however, discuss with the client the intolerable home situation and break down the problem to a more manageable focus that might be amenable to resolution.

The therapeutic process involves working with the client so that he understands the nature of his conflicts and how he contributes to them through self-deception. Then the counselor turns the problem around and asks the client what keeps him from using his strengths and capacities.

Even if the client sees his problem clearly and is highly motivated to solve it, there will be obstacles in his way. He will be thwarted by both conscious and unconscious resistances. On a conscious level, a client at times withholds information because of distrust, shame, or fear of rejection. A client may avoid looking at stressful topics because he is afraid that he cannot bear the pain. A conscious resistance, once recognized by the client as an unnecessary obstacle that is raised irrationally by him and not an inherent part of the situation, becomes readily accessible to the client for discussion. This is in contrast to an unconscious resistance, which involves "the instinctive opposition displayed towards any attempt to lay bare the unconscious."[1 (p 646)] Chapter 7 discusses typical clinical syndromes that are reflections of unconscious resistances and techniques for their management.

An example of unconscious resistance is intellectualizing. The client uses generalizations and inundates the counselor with words. The counselor realizes the client has touched a sore point that he would rather avoid. He recognizes that before the unconscious conflict that has generated this reaction can be explored, the client must first be made aware of the way in which he is attempting to hide something from himself and the counselor. Hence, the counselor is not impatient with this flood of words and knows that it is not easily stopped. The verbosity is an integral part of the client's coping mechanisms, and he is not going to give it up easily.

The first step with this or any other defense mechanism is for the counselor to respect it and attempt to understand it. The defense mechanisms serve to "protect the individual against dangers arising from his impulses or affects."[1 (p 178)] Depression, repression, reaction formation, isolation, undoing, projection, sublimation, denial, and so on, are regarded as defense mechanisms or problems that must be worked with as part of the entire therapeutic process and not as examples of untoward or uncooperative functioning.

The major initial goal of the therapeutic process is to interest and to assist the client in discovering how he as an individual works. The client's growing self-awareness and interest in his own thinking processes permit him to spend less time and energy judging, chastising, and punishing himself. He becomes increasingly able to accept himself and to change, within limits, parts of his thinking that are impeding his functioning. With greater objectivity and perspective the client can better handle his problems.

In the carefully designed situation of counselor and client, a most remarkable phenomenon, known as transference, occurs. In this process the client sees in the counselor features, real and imagined, of figures from his past, usually his parents. His responses to the counselor become distorted as they are affected and influenced by these earlier relationships. While the phenomenon of transference should be understood, the counselor need not analyze all such feelings nor interpret their origin. However, it is important to discuss gross negative transference feelings because they may block the client or cause resistance. Comments such as "You seem upset today," "How come you're so angry?" or "What is so irritating?" encourage the client to talk about negative feelings. Where the data allow it, a most useful move is to point out to the client the disproportion between the feelings and the event or non-event that seemed to provoke the anger. At such times the counselor needs to be alert to the possibility that the negative response may be to a real action of the counselor.

Transference feelings also occur in positive form. When a client is experiencing positive feelings toward the counselor, direct acknowledgment of these feelings by the counselor may be too anxiety-provoking for the client or may produce guilt and tension in him. It is necessary for the beginner to realize that these feelings are not really meant for him personally and do not require specific discussion. If the client expresses a positive feeling for the counselor, the counselor can tell the client that these same feelings can be experienced and expressed for friends or family.

A reverse phenomenon occurs when the counselor irrationally transfers to the client feelings from his previous life situation. Usually, recognition of these feelings by the counselor or sharing them with one's supervisor fosters self-awareness and neutralizes the situation. If a counselor finds himself becoming preoccupied or over-emotionally involved with a client, he must ask himself if he has lost his capacity to be objective and if it is wise for him to continue with this client.

The therapeutic process requires effective communication. Usually the initial material comes from the client who may begin by talking about what is easiest for him. If a client continually avoids painful, unpleasant, or difficult subjects, it becomes the task of the counselor to introduce these themes. Timing is important. Counselor and client together use their judgment to find the most reachable areas in order to exploit them for the learning that the client can relate to other situations.

Communication occurs at various levels. By listening to the client, the counselor judges or determines which area is the most fruitful to pursue and which conflicts are so entrenched that little would be accomplished by opening them up. In order for the counselor to differentiate between manifest and latent content, he must learn to listen. This requires practice and supervision. With manifest or conscious content the aim is to determine its coherence, consistency, relationship to mood, and repetitiousness. If the point of the manifest discussion is not clear, questions posed by the counselor can elicit more information and help to define what the client is getting at. There are ways to ask questions that enable the client to focus his thinking and make it easier for him to share his thoughts. Beginning a question with "Did," "How," "Where," "When," or "What" is more productive than beginning with "Why." "Why" usually leads to an intellectual response. Also, instead of helping the client to focus his thinking, it may connote to him disapproval or moralizing. He may interpret it as "Why did you do such a stupid thing?" Further, "Why" tends to imply to many people that knowing the motive is the important thing, but this is generally a form of intellectualizing rather than of understanding the process of how the mind works, which is the real goal.

MacKinnon and Michels point out that when the question "Why?" is asked, the client is bewildered. He "does not know why he became sick at this time or in this particular way or why he feels as he does."[2(p 19)] They stress the need for the interviewer to ask the client to elaborate or to provide details instead of asking why. To find out what inhibitions or conflicts interfere with the client's understanding, more useful questions are: "What got in the way?" "How did you decide it that way?" "What brought that about?" "Did you mind that?" "When did that happen?" and "How long has that been going on?" These questions lead to more readily accessible areas of investigation as a client searches his consciousness for clues to his own emotional functioning. (See the section on exploration, Chap. 3.)

Hidden meanings are harder to assess. Often the counselor "hears" the hidden messages by listening to the contradictions, inherent ambiguities, ambivalences, and conflicts in the client's statements. He notes the nonverbal, nonconscious intrusions and the relationship between these and the conscious statements. He tries to phrase his questions tactfully but in such a way that they provide information both about the manifest and latent content. When a client is not ready to answer searching questions, or when the subject is too painful and upsetting, the counselor recognizes and acknowledges this. He depends on the client to give him hints as to what is most available for discussion. Thus, he interferes as little as possible with what the client is saying until he has this sense of direction.

This book does not provide all the answers or techniques for interviewing. It is, instead, a guide to ways of thinking about and working with a person who is seeking treatment. There are no exact prescriptions for clients or for counselors. However, the client is entitled to believe that he is going to learn something useful from the interviews, that he will leave with increased clarity about himself and his living with other people.[3(p 18,19)]Does one try to use the client's language? Of course, when it permits the counselor to communicate more readily with the client, avoids misunderstanding, permits succinctness, and indicates that the client understood precisely what was meant. But, of course, *not* when such use might seem condescending or fail to supply the cognitive or intellectual structure that some counseling requires. The counselor listens and decides. He has an important responsibility, for it is the client who gets hurt when the counselor makes a mistake. However, the counselor who feels he can never err can also hurt the client. As long as the counselor is an ethical, humane person who accepts and understands his responsibility, most things can be worked out. No book on technique can supply those human qualities, but once they are there, a look at the ways counselors work and the principles that guide them may be of some use.

It is a premise of counseling that the intellectual and emotional understanding that the client works out within the therapeutic process will carry over to current and future life experiences. The therapeutic process provides a laboratory or a safe testing place for the client to study particular aspects about himself, with the assumption that what he learns will have general applicability outside of the counseling situation.

The techniques described in the following chapters will help beginners to get started and to feel more comfortable with clients. These methods are not just techniques but are also expressions of essential therapeutic principles. When we suggest that a counselor stop the interview on time—this does not mean that the client is cut off in mid-sentence or mid-paragraph—it is not because of a rigid preoccupation with exactness. Rather, it is because we want the client to be able to express his thoughts and feelings about the interview running over. Would the counselor be telling the client that he is special—and thus promising him favored treatment? Stopping on time is a technical suggestion, but the reason for it is a basic principle. In order for the counselor to work with the client towards accepting responsibility for himself, his thoughts, and his feelings and to develop an interest in how his mind works, the counselor needs techniques *and* an understanding of what lies behind them.

Even though the new counselor has a great deal to learn, he can begin to work as an effective interviewer. The interviewing experience itself will aid him as he gains in mastery of essential practical and theoretical principles.

REFERENCES

1. Hinsie LE, Campbell J: Psychiatric Dictionary, 3rd ed. New York, Oxford Univ Press, 1960
2. MacKinnon RA, Michels R: The Psychiatric Interview in Clinical Practice. Philadelphia, Saunders, 1971
3. Sullivan HS: The Psychiatric Interview. New York, Norton, 1954

2

THE THERAPEUTIC CONTEXT

As the therapeutic process unfolds, the role expectations of both the counselor and the client become more clearly defined. The relationship is voluntary (a few exceptions will be discussed later)—client and counselor come together as equals who have the same rights and privileges but not the same tasks as they work together on a common problem. The client presents his thoughts and feelings, with the conscious understanding that he will not be judged, disapproved of, laughed at, punished, or summarily rejected. Initially, this conscious knowledge about the situation does not go very deep.

The counselor's ability to listen to and accept what the client says and then, in this atmosphere of sincere interest, to show the client fresh ways of thinking about himself encourages the client to present himself more and more freely. The client sets his goals, but the counselor's comments contribute to the client's examination and review of his problems. This process may change the client's understanding and, consequently, his goals. Within this working partnership provided by the clinical interview, the participants assess and reassess the boundaries of their interaction—the rules of the game, if you will—how they select the structure they do, and where they expect it to take them.

In this working partnership the problem for the beginning counselor is to find a reasonable position between too little and too much concern for the client. The task becomes one of developing a balance between subjectivity and objectivity. Without objectivity the counselor lacks the psychological distance to do his part of the job, which is to find and describe the consistencies and patterns in the client's chaotic emotional responses so easily missed by the person himself.

Objectivity does not mean that the counselor is cold or dehumanized but rather that he pays attention to reality and points it out to the client as appropriate. Objectivity, however, without warmth and empathy may appear as a lack of interest to the client and will result in barren interaction. Most clients sense when they are treated like specimens rather than human beings and react by discontinuing the relationship. Some beginning counselors confuse the benevolent neutrality of the experienced therapist with the cold, disinterested stance of one unconcerned with counseling. Once the beginner experiences for himself the potential friendliness in objectivity, and is able to accept the difference between the counseling relationship and other social interactions, he is surprised by his earlier confusion.

Most counselors tend to lean too much in the direction of subjectivity, being excessively concerned and worried about the client. Some beginners experience this as a more desirable attitude since the only alternative they see is detachment. However, the stance can cause the counselor to behave like a philanthropist who graciously provides for the needy person, or an overly solicitous parent who smothers the child with giving. The client in this situation may develop a sense of obligation to the counselor, and he may wonder rightly what the counselor wants in return from him.

A counselor who is overly concerned or who overly identifies with his client may limit the therapeutic situation in other ways. Too much caring on the part of the counselor makes it hard for the client to express greed, envy, hate, or other emotions that he believes may disappoint or hurt the counselor. Overconcern or overcaring on the part of the counselor also reinforces the client's wish to place the counselor in a parental role. Even when the counselor maintains a correct, friendly objectivity, many clients will seek nurturance and evidence of caring inherent in the mothering role. The counselor who accepts this wished-for role increases the client's dependency wishes, encourages unreal expectations, and negates the potential for the client to discover that he really does not want the dependency he is seeking. In fact, his search for it erects constraints, increases internal conflict, and generally reduces his life space, so it is incumbent on the counselor to not go along with these wishes of the client. Other clients, looking for the bad or rejecting parent, will try to provoke the anger of the counselor, and if their tactics "succeed," this will interfere with an objective relationship. If the counselor is overinvolved, he is vulnerable to being provoked by the client's disappointing him or letting him down. Still other clients search for a friend, foe, lover, or omnipotent authority figure.

In the search for gratification and fulfillment of these wishes, clients unconsciously set up tests and traps for the counselor to fall into these roles. This is reflected in such comments as "If you really cared for me, you wouldn't go on vacation," "If you were really interested in my learning to socialize, you would teach me to dance," or "When are you going to cure my headaches?" (See the section on clarification, Chap. 3, for an explanation of these traps and ways of working them through.) If the counselor falls into these traps and attempts to fulfill the client's unrealistic expectations, he will defeat one of the purposes of the treatment, which is to permit the client to understand how the choice of such an unsuitable target for the fulfillment of these wishes interferes with his attaining them.

To deal with the client's overly dependent, angry, or critical feelings, the counselor needs to be aware that these reactions are not necessarily in response to his behavior nor to reality but instead may be rooted in the client's past and thus are the result of transference. (Transference is discussed in Chap. 1.) In almost all therapeutic interactions it is important that the counselor make clear to the client that the expression of such feelings is potentially "understandable" no matter how irrational or unreasonable the manifest content may seem. If the client has difficulty in expressing negative or positive feelings, the counselor will facilitate the client's understanding of this difficulty by looking into similar responses from the client's past.

Explanations from the past can also be overused. A counselor cannot automatically assume that the client's past has the answers. For one thing, when comparing and equating a reaction in the treatment situation with a response in the client's past, the counselor is assuming that the present response is patently irrational. To be on sure ground with such an assumption, the counselor must maintain a sharp eye and a questioning attitude toward his own behavior to see if it is a stimulus, even if only a minor one, to the client's reaction. A counselor, in common with the client, is a human being with emotions, such as fear, affection, annoyance, sexual desire, envy, and rage. The counselor must be constantly aware of the existence of these feelings within himself and of his human capacity for fallibility if he is to successfully prevent these feelings from interfering with the counseling. This constant assessment by the counselor of his own emotional state will help him to avoid being caught off guard by unexpected disturbances in the counseling situation.

Another reason that the past can be overstressed has to do with the goals of counseling. Of course, the basic goals of any treatment are set by the client. But the counselor knows that too great an interest in the past opens up for the client the hope that all of his life can be understood. Even formal psychoanalysis would dispute such an ambitious goal, and in more usual counseling situations, the counselor works with the client on the problem of selecting goals that seem more accessible. If the counselor at the same time digs incessantly into the past, he may confuse the client unless it is clear to both of them where this interest is headed.

The counselor's awareness of his own feelings and his acceptance of responsibility for controlling them sharply differentiate him from an ordinary social friend. Friends share their intimacies with each other, taking turns, in a sense, ventilating their feelings and offering temporary relief and support as they hear each other out. In counseling, the client is not expected to know the counselor's problems, let alone assist the counselor with them. Nor is the client expected to guide and correct the flow of the relationship. For these reasons, the client is free to deal with his own difficulties without any sense of burden about the feelings of the counselor.

If the counselor has to maintain his neutral role throughout, what prompts him to such hard work? The counselor's psychic returns from the relationship are of a different order from those in ordinary social relationships. He rejects the *usual* wish to be liked or to be gratified. How then does he maintain the place of human warmth in the therapeutic interaction? What, in other words, does he get out of it? It is important to note how frequently that question is asked in this discipline; it does not come up nearly as often in most other disciplines, such as law, electronics, or engineering. Because of the closeness and the frankness of the interaction in the counseling situation, people find it hard to believe that a counselor can settle for the same satisfactions that motivate other workers, such as earning a living, doing a good job, and feeling useful. What these people fail to understand is the fascination and inherent, if not overt, friendliness of the job. In the long run a good counselor can expect respect from his clients because of his ability to show them ways of looking at themselves that they themselves had missed. This can be a greatly satisfying human response. Each client, coming with his own challenges and lessons, permits the counselor to learn about the infinite complexity of human beings and human relationships. Despite the similarities, each person is essentially different from the next. From the knowledge that both counselor and client can learn something of value from the other can come a most satisfying experience for both.

In our view, the counselor through his objective stance presents himself as relatively invulnerable. No matter how personal or how intense the statements and the feelings of the client, the counselor treats them as manifestations of transference (see Chap. 1). The counselor's benevolent acceptance of these expressions and his attempts to make sense of them are part of his skill. Thus, the client has the freedom to express his emotions without fear. If a client misses sessions because of emotional turmoil or a vacation and desires to continue the counseling, he is responsible for those sessions. Should he remain silent out of a wish to punish the counselor, he soon realizes that it is his treatment that suffers. The situation is designed to make it clear that the impetus for the counseling is provided by the client's desire to discuss his problems, not the counselor's wish that he do so.

While the counselor's objectivity supports the crucial therapeutic neutrality, it becomes at the same time one of the most delicate therapeutic problems. Anyone who can accept without flinching feelings as powerful as the client experiences in his own deeper responses must appear either callous and uncaring or enormously powerful with the capacity to succor, to retaliate, or to judge. The client may experience the therapeutic neutrality as degrading or dehumanizing. "You are too weak and unimportant to have an effect on me," the counselor seems to be saying. The counselor, of course, knows all too well that he is not all-powerful, completely objective, or invulnerable. His capacity to react minimally to intense feelings of anger, love, or fear derives from his competence as a counselor and from his recognition that in the counseling situation he is only the temporary recipient of these feelings. Because of this minimal response, the client is able to see that his strong reactions to the therapeutic objectivity are part of the work—perhaps the most difficult, though potentially the most fruitful, part—and these reactions would not be available for discussion if the counselor were to become too involved.

As we see one-to-one interviewing, the counselor is expected to be objective and to remain so. He is committed to the study of an individual case, rather than to a system, such as a group, a ward, a family, or a social stratum. He values the shared work of the counseling—two people working together toward understanding—and avoids viewing the client as seeking "help," which bestows weakness on the person in need of help and strength on the person with this help to offer. Although he knows the importance of nonverbal messages and values frank emotionalism and irrationality, he relies on verbal communication and, eventually, rationality. He is aware of the important message about his values that is conveyed by his generally neat appearance and carefully selected surroundings and his avoidance of a deviant or disruptive social atmosphere, and he does not impose these values on his clients. His conventionality is unlikely to indicate to the client a special ax to grind, which the client might interpret from unconventionality, and does not necessarily reflect the counselor's personal positions in his private life.

Thus, the working model, the therapeutic context, consists of two people who are equal but who have different tasks. One of them supplies the subjectivity, the other the objectivity, and this stance of relative equality can always be reintroduced as the base of the relationship if the client loses sight of his goals.

3
TECHNIQUES OF INTERVIEWING

THE WORKING RELATIONSHIP

Counseling interviews must be carried on in an atmosphere of openness in which the client realizes that he has the opportunity and is encouraged to understand and work out his problems. If a counselor takes too literally a description of his position as a "helper," he will not be able to conduct an open, interactive interview. As discussed earlier, a counselor's ready offer "to help" is likely to mislead the client into thinking that the counselor has special advice or magical solutions to offer, and it also gratifies the client's wish to be reactive or passive instead of doing his share of the work. The beginning counselor should not feel that it is his task to solve the client's problems. He will be of more service to his client if he engages him to work in his own behalf.

Thus, it is necessary for the counselor to keep a clear vision of treatment as a mutual task in which counselor and client work together toward an understanding and resolution of the client's difficulties. In other words, the counselor and the client have a *working relationship* in which they establish together a working agreement or understanding of their respective jobs and the corresponding responsibilities and privileges. The beginner is advised to avoid the word "help" and to substitute, instead, the phrase "work with you" as he begins to develop a working relationship with the client.

In order to promote an open atmosphere, the counselor begins the relationship by "starting where the client is."[3(p 36)] This means that the counselor encourages the client to talk about what is on *his* mind. Such questions as "How are things?" "What's been going on?" "Where do you wish to begin?" "Where shall we start?" or "What do you want to work on?" encourages the client to discuss what he considers to be important. Once the client begins to talk, the counselor's capacity to accept and the client's ability to understand what is being presented further set the tone of the relationship.

The counselor, by showing interest in and empathy for the client, communicates to him both verbally and nonverbally that the interview is client-centered. To keep the focus on the client, the counselor listens to the client's comments and observes his facial and body expressions, concentrating on both the latent and the manifest content of the verbal discussion as well as on the nonverbal cues.

> A counselor had several interviews with Ms. Webber, who was seeking help with her marital relationship. Her initial concern centered on the constant bickering between her and her husband and its effect on their three daughters. During the first sessions Ms. Webber talked about the stormy marriage, focusing mainly on the interaction between her and her husband. During the sixth interview, she mentioned that she was quite worried about her oldest daughter, who had been shutting herself up in her room every night. The counselor asked for more details about the daughter's behavior, but he also asked Ms. Webber about her reactions to this behavior, with such questions as "How are you handling it?" "Are you commenting about it, or are you ignoring it?" "What ideas do you have about it?" These exploratory questions related to the client's reactions forced the client to talk more about herself. They also showed the counselor's interest in and concern for the client.

ESTABLISHING THE WORKING AGREEMENT

Practical arrangements such as the frequency and length of interviews, the fee, the different roles of client and counselor, and the extent of the client's conscious or unconscious commitment to work toward understanding himself must be settled to some degree before the counseling arrangement gets under way.

Obviously, these matters are reviewed frequently and often become a focus of the counseling. Goals, in particular, once negotiated, can be renegotiated within the framework of the client's wishes and the counselor's understanding of their mutual functioning within the therapeutic context.

Each party during this early discussion of rights and responsibilities has a rare opportunity to state his position. The counselor can say directly what services can be provided within the framework of the agency's functions and his view of his role and tasks. The client can identify his problems and express his hopes and face the difference between these hopes and the realities of counseling. By discussing how they may work together, the counselor indicates the limits of the situation and begins his task of pointing out reality wherever necessary.

EXPLORATION

It is essential to "explore" what the client's perception of his situation is and what his expectations are so that the client may understand for himself what he is seeking or what is troubling him. The counselor's nonverbal cues, such as a nod, a smile, silence, or a questioning look, are an indication to the client that the counselor is listening. The counselor inquires about the client's problem in an open-ended and nonjudgmental fashion.

The asking of evocative questions is basic to the ongoing process of the interview as it stimulates and encourages the client to think in new ways about himself. When the counselor asks for additional information, the client is encouraged to provide more details, which often open up the feelings connected to the situation and prepare the client for greater understanding.

As discussed in Chapter 1, there are ways to ask questions that enable the client to share his thoughts; it is best not to begin a question with "Why," which may be interpreted as judging or may lead to an intellectual response, but, instead, to begin with "Did," "How," "Where," "When," or "What." The following comments and questions are samples: "Tell me more, I didn't understand." "Could you explain that further?" "What do you mean?" "I'm not sure I understand what you're trying to say." "How do you explain what happened?" "How did that happen?" "When did that happen?" "What's that about?" "What do you understand about this?" "What are your ideas on that?" "How come you left home?" "What made you leave home?"

If a client describes a problem, the counselor asks for specific examples regarding the nature of the problem; that is, he is asking the client what really bothers him, what he argues about, what makes him feel helpless in his situation. When a client says, "My husband makes me angry," the counselor asks, "What does he do or say that makes you angry?"

Examples of exploration include: The Stewarts came to a clinic to discuss their marital difficulties. Ms. Stewart had accused her husband of being an alcoholic and blamed their problems on his drinking. The counselor, who was faced with the task of exploring the situation without alienating either of them, asked for more details about how the marriage had been going and what the couple saw as their problems. He asked what shifts and changes there had been that might have affected the relationship, such as work pressures, problems in the extended family network, and so on. As the couple answered these questions, they began to see some stresses in their marriage that they had not recognized before. They could then decide about how they wanted to proceed.

Mr. Brush, age 32, came to treatment for the first time. The counselor began the session by asking, "What brings you here?" The client stated that his wife had accused him of being short-tempered, hostile, and uninterested in sex because of the long hours he worked. He did not feel this to be a serious problem and only agreed to see a counselor because his wife had insisted that he do so. This was a delicate situation for the counselor because Mr. Brush was not well motivated and could easily be put off. The counselor dealt with the situation by taking it up directly. He asked Mr. Brush how he felt about being pushed into counseling by his wife. The counselor went on and asked if this was something new or if Mr. Brush found himself being pushed into other situations by his wife. He also asked how long this had been going on. In this way the counselor followed the principles of starting "where the client is" and stimulated him to see the situation from a different perspective.

Inquiry into Embarrassing Subjects

Often the beginning counselor needs to discuss subjects that he feels are difficult or embarrassing. The client may also feel uncomfortable about discussing certain topics. Almost any counseling has moments that are embarrassing for either the client or the counselor, or both. There is no set subject matter that may cause embarrassment, and one can expect surprises here as elsewhere in counseling. It may be as difficult for some people to talk about success as it is easy for others, and the same holds true for practically any subject. Perhaps the only universal factor is the fundamental irrationality, in either person, that stimulates the embarrassment.

There is a tendency for beginners to avoid or shut off topics that are difficult for them. Similarly, clients avoid things about which they are embarrassed or uncomfortable. What makes a subject embarrassing depends on many factors including the upbringing and personality structure of the person involved. What the client may regard as a strength, the counselor may regard as a problem, and vice versa. When an embarrassing topic is introduced, regardless of how it comes up, it may be important to keep it in mind and explore it for the client's better understanding of his conflicts. This may be very difficult for a beginner, who may himself be shy about "touchy subjects." However, the counselor's inability to be open and frank about such subjects increases the client's feelings of discomfort and may abort the possibility of useful discussion.

Finances.   Frequently, one of the subject areas that is most difficult or embarrassing is money or financial status. When a beginner has to discuss fee setting, he often finds it awkward, possibly because of his own doubts about his worth. A client may find it difficult to discuss finances when he has been successful. It can be just as difficult for an affluent man to tell the details of his accomplishments as it is for an unsuccessful man to reveal his financial limitations and failures in earning money.

Obtaining information about a client's salary or income can be an awesome task for the beginner. Often, the higher the education, intellectual level, or social class of the client, the more difficult it is for beginners to inquire about financial details. Sometimes it is easier to ask general questions, such as "Will your salary cover this?" or "Does your insurance pay for counseling?" A way of proceeding in a less specific manner is to ask whether the client has any outstanding debts. As with any potentially embarrassing subject, the counselor needs to be sensitive about his client's attitudes toward money. It will be easier for a client to be open about such subjects if the counselor is comfortable asking the question and provides a clear rationale for the necessity of sharing the information.

Sex. Another difficult topic may be sex. Again, it can be as difficult to describe successful sexual experiences as unsuccessful ones.

> Ms. Sand, age 27, was in counseling for several months before she mentioned her concern about her sex life with her husband. When the counselor attempted to explore what it was she was actually worried about, Ms. Sand was blocked and could not say what was on her mind. The counselor told her that whatever sexual practices a couple mutually agree on as enjoyable are acceptable. Subsequent to this, Ms. Sand brought out her husband's wish for cunnilingus and her fear that this was an indication that he had serious problems. The counselor reminded her that it was up to the two people involved as to what was agreeable and urged her to decide on the grounds of mutual pleasure.

Some situations involving sex can be embarrassing or awkward for the counselor, such as with clients who are sexually attracted to their counselor and ask directly or indirectly for some degree of satisfaction.

> Mr. Martin, age 42, had recently been separated from his wife and was now living alone. He was seeing a counselor because he was depressed and functioning poorly at work. During one of the sessions Mr. Martin revealed to his young female counselor that he had been thinking a great deal about her over the weekend and wanted her to go out to dinner with him. He was afraid he was becoming impotent and was hopeful she would help him with his problem. He felt certain that he would be successful with her and wanted to show her that he was still a man. The counselor felt very uncomfortable, but managed to acknowledge her awareness of Mr. Martin's loneliness and worries about himself. She pointed out that it was unrealistic to change the counseling relationship into a social one as that would defeat its purpose. She suggested, instead, that he use the therapeutic relationship to understand what got in his way socially and sexually so that he could feel more comfortable in his usual social situation. They were then able to explore his inhibitions about meeting women and relating to them sexually.

Some clients, especially adolescents, may ask their counselors specific questions about their sex life. It is not appropriate to tell the client such intimate details (see the section Personal Questions, Chap. 5). In responding a counselor can explain that the issue is not information about his private life but, instead, the client's concern about the information.

Forced Marriage. Often in obtaining history the counselor picks up clues about a client's background such as a forced marriage due to pregnancy. While the client may not want to discuss the issue in detail, the counselor may find it necessary to inquire about the circumstances of the marriage.

> A counselor asked his client, Mr. Abbot, age 50, about the circumstances of his marriage. In response, Mr. Abbot appeared embarrassed, squirmed in his chair, cleared his throat, flushed, and obviously found it difficult to discuss the marriage. Although he didn't know the reason, the counselor recognized that this was a "charged" subject for the client. He knew also that it was important to discuss it even though Mr. Abbot was uncomfortable in doing so. Mr. Abbot then told the counselor that he had always been embarrassed about giving his marriage date because his wife was pregnant prior to their marriage and this was still a sore subject between them.

Homosexuality. Although homosexuality is not as forbidden a subject as it once was, many clients still find the topic difficult to discuss.

> Ms. Barber went to see a counselor because she was having problems with her 15-year-old son. During the initial interview the counselor asked Ms. Barber what some of her son's difficulties had been. Ms. Barber said that her son was having trouble in school and that his grades were slipping. He was also keeping late hours and never told her where he was going or with whom. She indicated that there were other things she was worried about but preferred not to go into them. The counselor appreciated her reticence but suggested that she be open about these matters as their work together could not be meaningful unless they were discussed. Ms. Barber then started to cry, saying that her son was a homosexual and she thought it was such a disgrace. The counselor asked her to explain what homosexual meant, not only to obtain information, but for the client's education to the fact that homosexuality is often a grab-bag word with more shock effect than substantial meaning. The counselor also recognized Ms. Barber's unhappiness and disappointment and suggested that these were reactions that they could look at together.

Family Secrets. Sometimes people are extremely self-conscious about family secrets that do not even directly concern the client or the obvious immediate family. Such secrets can lead to confusion if they are not tactfully discussed.

> Ms. Webber, age 38, consulted a counselor regarding her marital relationship. She said that she was thinking of leaving her husband because he was more attached to his mother than to her and their five children. In fact, he was very devoted to his whole family, and they all counted on him. During one interview, she brought up her concern that her 11-year-old son would grow up to be like her husband's brother. When the counselor asked Ms. Webber what her brother-in-law was like, her eyes darted downward, and she said, "Oh, he's just no good." The counselor asked what she meant by "no good." Ms. Webber further avoided the question by saying, "He's just a rotten apple." The counselor told the client that he was aware that Ms. Webber was covering something up and that it would be better if she could share what was on her mind. Ms. Webber then confided that her brother-in-law was currently serving a jail sentence for murder. She went on to say that her husband was very embarrassed about this and had told her to keep it a secret. However, she felt much better after talking about it.

Frequently, a family or a particular family member decides that an illness or a handicap must be kept secret.

> Mr. Harvey, age 48, entered counseling because of depression and inability to hold a job for more than a few months. In exploring Mr. Harvey's family background the counselor asked for his father's occupation. The client launched into a long discussion of how difficult his father was to get along with and how his bad temper made everyone in his family afraid of him, Mr. Harvey included. The counselor wondered how Mr. Harvey's father got along at work with such a bad temper and was told by the client that this was not a problem at work. When the counselor went back to the initial question of Mr. Harvey's father's occupation, the client answered that his father had worked only sporadically. The counselor then asked who had supported the family. Mr. Harvey looked sad and said that the family had been on welfare and that his father had been in and out of hospitals until his death. When the counselor questioned Mr. Harvey about the circumstances of his father's death, he reluctantly confided that his father had committed suicide in a mental hospital. Mr. Harvey then told the counselor that he had always been ashamed of his father's illness and did not like to tell anyone about it and that he often worried that he might end up like his father.

In the above examples the counselor had to take an active role of probing and directly questioning the client in order to explore embarrassing topics. There are clients, however, who easily volunteer information about potentially embarrassing topics, and the discussion flows easily.

CLARIFICATION

As defined by Dr. Edward Bibring, clarification refers to the process by which material which is conscious or preconscious and readily accessible is called to the client's attention.[1] (p 755) The counselor clarifies when he tells the client his observations and perceptions as to the order and sequence of what the client is presenting. Clarification is only possible after exploring with the client his view of his problems, his recollections, his behavior, his thoughts, ideas, worries, fears, and reactions. With this background the counselor puts together the emerging patterns of behavior, repetitions, conflicts, consistencies, interactional problem areas, and inhibitions. The counselor endeavors to clarify the issues for the client by presenting his observations to him for further examination.

Mr. Stone, age 40, was in counseling because of depression following the death of his wife one year earlier. He was also concerned about his son, who had required hospitalization for psychiatric care. At one point his son, who was suicidal, had threatened to leave the hospital. Mr. Stone was then asked to agree to a petition for a court order to commit his son. His reaction was to refuse. The counselor was puzzled by Mr. Stone's response and wondered what caused him to be so reluctant to protect his son? The counselor asked Mr. Stone what had prevented him from going along with the hospital's recommendation, and also pointed out that Mr. Stone seemed tense and agitated when discussing this recommendation. When the client became aware of his agitation, he revealed his disturbing past experience at age 16 when his own brother became psychotic and was committed to a mental institution by a court order. The counselor's observation about Mr. Stone's tenseness allowed the client to explore his hidden feelings, which led him to a better understanding of the conflict he was having about his son.

WORKING THROUGH

A client may mention, identify, or recognize a problem. However, acknowledgment is not a resolution. In order to work a problem through, or be able to manage it differently, the client examines and reexamines the issues. Through reviewing the details of past experiences, fears, wishes, worries, and so on, and approaching the conflict from different vantage points, he will begin to see the irrational origins of the conflicts. In this way, he will come to learn and understand more about himself and eventually be able to transfer that learning to new conflicts outside the therapeutic situation. The process of review and re-review of the material may appear to be extremely repetitious; however, the reviews are often accompanied by the client's newly gained insights into the issue. And it is necessary to examine in a step-by-step fashion the genesis and repeated occurrences of any intense emotional conflict. Intellectual recognition is the first step, but emotional acceptance evolves only through the understanding that comes from repeated review of the issue.

Learning new adaptive responses to situations that previously have brought about irrational responses is difficult and time-consuming. In fact, few people achieve perfect results. At best, a client will build up some understanding about his reactions that will make it possible for him to cope better with present and future problems.

Ms. Jones, age 34, sought treatment because she had either been fired from or had left eight jobs in two years and realized something was wrong. She reported the dates and places where she had worked and named the source of the conflict in each place: too much work; not enough work; it was boring; the boss did not like her; the other employees were too competitive; her mother had been ill and she was needed at home; and so forth. Initially she blamed all her difficulties on the environment in which she found herself and resisted the idea that something within herself was in her way. The counselor explored her mother's sickness and Ms. Jones's relationship with her family. He also explored the nature of the jobs and the details of each experience, in an attempt to get Ms. Jones to see the links between each job problem.

Each time she recounted her story, she was able to give more details and began to see a pattern emerging wherein she had initiated or caused all her job terminations. She began to realize she was seeking rejection. Whenever she lost her job, she imagined that her mother would take her in and be especially attentive. From her childhood she recalled that she felt she only got her mother's attention when she was in some sort of difficulty. She recognized that she caused her work problems and saw the ways in which she sabotaged herself. The achievement by Ms. Jones of this intellectual understanding did not eliminate her problem with keeping a job. But instead of simply leaving a job or getting fired, she began to repeatedly struggle with ("work through") these conflicts at work.

ENVIRONMENTAL MODIFICATION

Instead of exploring only the emotional content of the material, the counselor's and client's goal may be to bring about a change in the client's life situation.[2 (p 231)] This effort to modify the external environment works better if the client is able to take direct action for himself. However, when this is beyond the client's control, or when the counselor's pressures on the client are more likely to result in change, then the counselor intervenes in the situation.[4 (p 220-221)]

The counselor explores with the client the reasons for his request, his circumstances, the background of the problem, and the attempts he has made to solve the problem. When the client and the counselor both agree on the need for change, an understanding is reached as to how the change will be made and who will take action.

Ms. Porter had been receiving government support for her two young children. She told the counselor that she wanted help in obtaining a job because she needed more money. The counselor asked the client what her thoughts were about getting a job in order for them to review together the background and motivation that had led the client to seek counseling. They considered the advisability of contacting a housekeeper or babysitting service and discussed the possibility of obtaining assistance from other agencies. After the client understood her request and could assess its validity, the client and the counselor came to an agreement as to what action was necessary and who should take it.

Mr. Barry was referred to a counselor for assistance in arranging for psychiatric hospitalization for his 72-year-old mother, whom he had recently brought to the emergency ward of a general hospital. She had many somatic complaints and talked openly of her wish to join her husband, who had died from a heart attack three weeks earlier. Mr. Barry was quite upset by the doctor's recommendation for psychiatric hospitalization, and when he seemed reluctant to follow through on it, he was referred to the counselor.

On inquiring into Mr. Barry's distress, the counselor learned that Mr. Barry had hoped that medication would relieve his mother's symptoms. Also, he felt guilty about all the years he had ignored her and felt that he should make it up to her. He was concerned about the stigma of having a relative in a mental institution and worried about how he would tell his wife and children that his mother was "crazy." In reviewing with Mr. Barry his worries and concerns, his fears and distorted attitudes became apparent to him. Mr. Barry began to recognize the difference between the external reality of his mother's condition and his emotional conflicts. When some of his personal concerns became more conscious and separated from the issue of his mother's current illness, Mr. Barry was better able to focus on his mother's needs and agreed to have her hospitalized.

PERSONAL OPINIONS AND ADVICE

Generally speaking, beginners do not give advice, as usually they do not have any certainty about what is truly better for the client. In particular, counselors, whether they are beginners or experienced practitioners, should refrain from offering opinions on spiritual or moral issues. While the intent may be "to help" the client, such opinions frequently convey other meanings to the client. A counselor may be tempted to offer someone afraid of death the hope of an afterlife, or to point out the advantages of democracy or freedom to a member of a totalitarian gang. However, such information, no matter how well meant, puts the counselor in the position of being an omniscient, preaching, paternalistic figure and prevents the development of a working relationship. The client may ask the counselor about his ideology because the client is unsure of his own and thinks the counselor's would be a better one to follow. If the counselor freely gives this information to the client, he will be fostering the client's belief that the counselor has all the solutions to his problems.

There are various issues about which a client might seek the counselor's advice or opinion or ask what he would do in the client's situation, such as divorce, marriage, job or school choice, and living arrangements. When this arises, the counselor points out that the decisions rest with the client and that what the counselor would do is not the issue. The subsequent disappointment and rejection that the client may feel when the counselor withholds his personal opinion do not alter the principles. It is useful to discuss the client's feelings about not getting what he wanted.

Occasionally, a client will be in a situation that will warrant the advice of the counselor. In these cases the counselor and the client must have established a relationship in which the client understands the counselor's purpose in giving him advice and is able to use the advice constructively.

Ms. Parsons sought help from a children's agency when she considered placing her nine-year-old son in a foster home because of his temper tantrums, overeating, and constant demands for attention. When the counselor inquired about the ways Ms. Parsons had attempted to cope with her son's behavior, Ms. Parsons revealed that she had allowed the boy to sleep with her so that he would feel she was giving him attention. Because the counselor felt this sleeping arrangement was too stimulating and provocative for the son, he told Ms. Parsons that it would be better if she did not let the boy sleep with her. Ms. Parsons was relieved by the advice since she had felt uncomfortable with her attempted solution. The client and the counselor then proceeded to discuss alternative ways of dealing with the problem.

[handwritten margin note: CRITICAL ADVICE -]

A 19-year-old student sought counseling about his decision to get married. He told the counselor that he had felt lonely all his life and that now he had found the perfect girl. This client was not interested in counseling. What he really wanted was permission to go ahead and get married. He had only gone to the counselor because his father had threatened to cut him off financially if he got married and he would probably have to drop out of school and go to work. If the counselor approved of his getting married, the client felt his father would approve also. The counselor suggested that the client postpone the precipitous marriage while they worked on the client's feelings of loneliness. The young man refused. He did not have a sufficiently developed relationship with the counselor and felt the counselor was talking like his father and not being objective.

PRAISE

As with opinions and advice, a beginner avoids giving praise. The client may interpret praise as false reassurance or lack of real understanding on the part of the counselor.

Ms. Smith, age 24, consulted a counselor at an adult psychiatric clinic. Since her boyfriend had left her four days earlier, she had been feeling worthless and despondent. She had not been eating or sleeping, and she felt ugly and certain that no one would ever care for her again. When the counselor told Ms. Smith that she was pretty and therefore had nothing to worry about, Ms. Smith felt that the counselor was insensitive and lacking in understanding.

Mr. Webb sought counseling because of his problems at work. He was also concerned about his wife, who had become very depressed when their youngest child entered kindergarten. During the second session he reported that his wife had gotten a job. Without asking or waiting for the client's reaction to this, the counselor enthusiastically told the client how pleased he was by that news. Several sessions later Mr. Webb started to talk about how upset he was by the fact that his wife was working. He said that she had not made adequate arrangements for the care of their children and that she was still depressed and refused to seek counseling. He had wanted to talk about his feelings earlier but had held back as long as he could because he felt the counselor would be disappointed in him for not being happy about his wife's job.

REFERENCES

1. Bibring E: Psychoanalysis and the dynamic psychotherapies. J Am Psychoanal Assoc 2:745–770, 1954
2. Bibring GL: Psychiatric principles in casework. J Soc Casework 30:230–235, 1949
3. Garrett A: Interviewing: Its Principles and Methods, 2nd ed. New York, Family Service Association of America, 1972
4. Hollis F: Casework: A Psychosocial Therapy. New York, Random House, 1964

4
PARAMETERS OF THE INTERVIEW

ROLE EXPECTATIONS OF THE CLIENT
AND THE COUNSELOR

A client comes to a counseling appointment full of fears, anxieties, and tensions comparable to the strain one experiences in any new situation. Everyone is familiar with the fear of being sent to the principal's office for the first time, taking a driving test for the first time, going on the first college interview, and the first job interview. Probably everyone has experienced sweaty palms, concern over appearance, apprehension about what to say or how to act in first meetings. These are experiences common to both the beginning interviewer and interviewee. While the therapeutic situation is similar in some ways to a new business or social situation, it is different in that in the therapeutic situation the client is expected to answer personal questions without the usual social subterfuges and the counselor is expected to maintain a careful objectivity.

Through the years, cultural and societal attitudes have influenced the client's expectations of psychological counseling. The client's own socioeconomic and cultural background and intellectual skills may also have a bearing on his view of counseling. These background factors often offer clues to the nature of the client's expectations of the counselor and counseling and will influence the treatment planning. The counselor on his part assumes that the client has the capacity to benefit from treatment. The mere act of accepting him as a client is an indication of the counselor's faith in the client's ability to work on his problems. Basing his practice on an established body of knowledge grounded in psychological theory and methods of treatment fosters the counselor's feeling of competence and enhances the therapeutic process. Unfortunately, not every client responds, and not every case is a success, but at least the counselor has approached the problem to the best of his ability and has applied his knowledge of psychological theory and method.

Most beginning counselors worry about the client's reaction to him as well as his ability to function adequately and appropriately. The beginner is often a student and is also concerned about what his teachers or supervisors will think of him. In the interview situation, the beginning interviewer can be compared to the principal, the admissions officer, the employer, that is, the person who is expected to be the expert. Because the interviewer is being trained in interpersonal relations and personality problems, he does have special knowledge from which the client hopes to benefit. As in any business transaction, the client is hiring a service and has the right to expect something useful in return for the fee. From the counselor's point of view, "The interviewer must be sure that the other person is getting something out of it, that his expectation of improving himself (as he may put it), or getting a better job, or of attaining whatever has motivated him in undergoing the interview, gets encouragement."[2](p 17)

There are certain considerations that if thought out beforehand and then kept in mind may help to allay some of the counselor's initial anxiety.

The Counselor's Appearance

The client's ability to relate to the counselor may be influenced by the counselor's appearance. If a young counselor accentuates his youth by extreme or sloppy clothes, makeup, or hairdo, the client may question his or her maturity. This could undermine the counselor's status as a competent professional person in the eyes of the client. Dressing in a provocative manner may call attention to the counselor and may stimulate discussion or personal thoughts about him. This may interfere with the counselor's objective of focusing on the client.[1(p 13)]

Acceptable dress and hair styles change depending on what is in vogue. Whereas beards and long hair for men and pantsuits for women may not have been acceptable a few years ago, they have recently been in style. However, some people are very suspicious and would have difficulty relating to a man with an unkempt beard or a woman with high-fashion clothing. It is sometimes necessary for the interviewer to make a compromise between his personal taste and the conventions of the setting in which he is employed.

Seating Arrangements

It is a good idea to arrange adequate seating and specific organization of the chairs in advance. Although some interviewers prefer to sit behind a desk, this is not necessary. It is up to the counselor to decide where he would feel most comfortable and most at ease. In some situations the desk may be a barrier between the interviewer and the client, whereas in others it can be used effectively to add distance where closeness is part of the problem. Traditionally, counselors have positioned themselves behind a desk. This was a way for the counselor to keep some distance from the client in order to feel more professional. In fact, sitting behind a desk does not necessarily achieve distance or maintain professionalism. Nowadays many counselors arrange their offices with the desk out of the way and with the seating more casual. As the counselor develops skills in interviewing techniques, he will feel more comfortable wherever he sits. The client is more apt to feel that the counselor is interested in and concerned about him if the office is arranged with thought and consideration, i.e., with comfortable chairs.

> Mr. Prince, age 37, entered treatment with a long history of inability to function at a job despite strong motivation for success in this area. Although he had expected a magical solution to his problem, he did make a commitment to work on his conflicts. This client, who was unmarried and had never been able to establish a close relationship with anyone, usually sat in the chair farthest removed from the counselor.

Ms. O'Brien, who had a very close, symbiotic tie with her mother, elected to sit in the chair closest to the counselor. The counselor understood this gesture as a function of her unconscious wishes to be close to the counselor in the same way that she felt close to her mother, from whom she had so much trouble separating.

These examples indicate that where the client elects to sit may be of diagnostic significance. Therefore, giving the client a choice in seating may offer clues about the client's ways of relating to people.

While this book is not geared specifically to interviewing families as a unit, it is noteworthy that family counselors customarily sit among the family members, without the intrusion of a desk. This enables the counselor to more quickly become involved with the family as a unit, and the family can more easily feel the counselor's presence and participation in working on their problems.

Entering the Office

Upon entering the office the client usually chooses the chair he wishes to sit in. Some clients experience a conflict about where to sit and ask for direction. A response of "Wherever you like" is an indication that the client can make his own choice and lets him know from the outset that the counselor does not have all the answers. Telling a client where to sit may confirm his wishes that the counselor will tell him what to do. (See Chap. 1, The Therapeutic Process, p 1.) Occasionally there may be a client who is so extremely anxious that he is unable to make a seating choice, in which case the counselor is forced to point out a chair.

If there is a specific place to hang coats and hats, the counselor may tell the client where it is. Occasionally, a client may sit huddled in his coat. He ought to be allowed this option without more than an initial question asking him if he would like to hang up his coat. However, this alerts the counselor that the client is anxious and probably very reluctant to expose himself in any way.

Ms. Kelly, age 55, usually chose not to remove her coat throughout the interview. She was a very dependent, infantile woman who deprecated herself verbally and was quick to view others' comments as criticism. Her initial explanation for not removing her coat was that she felt "too cold." This continued through eight interviews. At the beginning of the ninth interview she removed her coat, stating that it had become warmer in the office. Although Ms. Kelly did not give a realistic explanation for taking off her coat, she did become more open in expressing angry feelings toward her husband and children. She also began to reveal more about herself and to look at some of her feelings of worthlessness. Because Ms. Kelly never brought up the subject of the significance of keeping her coat on, the counselor decided not to mention it. It is possible that if the counselor had commented on it, Ms. Kelly would have taken his remark as a criticism rather than as a therapeutic issue for discussion.

Mr. Brown, age 38, was a very isolated person. He worried about his sexual inadequacies and sat huddled in his coat, complaining of the cold. His feeling cold provided the opening for the counselor to inquire if the chill was in the office or in their relationship. Mr. Brown then said that he was disappointed in the counselor because his symptoms had not been relieved and he felt put off.

Forms of Address for the Client

In traditional clinical settings, the usual approach is to address a client in his late adolescent years or older as Mr. Smith or Ms. Jones. A formal address makes explicit the professional nature of the relationship. In addition, addressing the client in a formal manner stresses to him that the counselor regards him as an adult who is expected to behave as one.

If the client asks to be called by his first name, the counselor can acknowledge that the client's request is an understandable one. The counselor then has three choices in dealing with such a request: (1) He may decide to go along with the request; (2) he may decide to keep it open for further discussion; or (3) he may decide not to honor the request, explaining that for this client last names are preferable. An agreement in the form of address between counselor and client is often seen as tentative and may be the subject of later discussion and possible revision.

James Peterson, age 27, was working with an older female counselor. He was very insulted when she called him Mr. Peterson. He was used to being called Jimmy and despised the family name, which was prominent and well known. He felt that he could not live up to the family expectations. He sought counseling because of severe depression and inability to take on the responsibility of marriage. The counselor felt that forcing the issue and insisting on calling the client by his last name would have alienated him to such a point that he might not have returned. Instead, she asked him how other people addressed him. Through this exploration, she learned that he encouraged people to think of him as Jimmy so that he could maintain what he regarded as a weak, childish position. It became obvious that his last name was symbolic of the adult status that he had long feared. The counselor recognized that the client's last name represented a complicated conflict with his father, and she elected to call him James. She pointed out that by calling himself Jimmy, he was being self-demeaning.

Richard Pratt, age 32, had been hospitalized for years and had been called Dickie by all the staff. By addressing him this way the staff members were unintentionally infantilizing him, which he found very gratifying and apparently the staff did also. When a new counselor was introduced and called him by his last name, Mr. Pratt was very angry initially. He pointed out that the other staff members, whom he regarded as his friends, called him Dickie. In his desire to also regard his counselor as a friend, which was his preferred way of relating to people, he wished to be called by his first name. In this instance, the counselor told Mr. Pratt that he thought the first name issue might be a conflict and indicated that he and the client were equals working together on his problems. By leaving the issue open, the counselor was encouraging Mr. Pratt to think over the feelings that went into such expectations.

Janet Dodd had three children and was separated from her husband. She entered treatment after a depression and psychotic decompensation. She was unable to cope with the responsibilities of being a mother and a wife. When the counselor called her Ms. Dodd, she began to cry and asked to be called by her first name. Prior to this, Ms. Dodd had been very unemotional and had maintained a high degree of denial about her conflicts and problems. The counselor pointed out that in calling her by her last name intense feelings had surfaced in her and forced her to acknowledge her conflict of taking on the responsibilities of marriage and motherhood. Continuing to call her by her last name fostered the therapeutic process.

How to Get Started

Although clients have a great deal on their minds and will usually begin talking soon after they arrive, the beginner often worries about how he will get the client to talk. Once the initial greeting has taken place, the counselor shares the responsibility of starting the interview. If the client is quiet at the first interview, such questions as "What brings you here?" or "How did your problems begin?" sometimes get things started. If the client is unresponsive, the interviewer can tell the client what he already knows about him or what he understands the purpose of the meeting to be. If the client has been transferred and has seen another counselor previously, either briefly or over a long period of time, the new counselor might comment that he has been talking to the other counselor or has read his record and knows a little about the situation. When a client has seen another counselor, it is important to ask the client about that experience— what it was about, how he got along with the counselor, and if he found it useful.

If the client says that all the information is in his record or that he has already told the previous worker everything, then the present counselor can point out that even though it may be annoying to repeat oneself, he would like to know from the client what brought him there. The counselor can also explain that reading a record or getting the facts from another person is not the same as hearing about the situation in the client's own words. The client needs to be told that his formulation of his problems and the way they affect him are more relevant than what is in the record. When a counselor is confronted with a client's statement, "Haven't you read my record?" there are various ways of replying. It may be useful to say, "Yes, but we want most of all to think about your experience of the situation," or "we need to understand how the situation has been affecting you—your life, your feelings, your activities, and your welfare."[3(p 198)]

There are times when requests for information should be deferred until the client brings up the particular issue or the counselor finds a more opportune moment to raise the issue after the relationship has been established.

Ms. Robbins, age 45, entered counseling for the second time in order to work out her feelings toward her husband, who had become a drug addict. When the counselor inquired about her previous treatment, Ms. Robbins revealed that she had terminated treatment prematurely because she could not tolerate what she interpreted as her counselor's excessive interest in her sex life. She felt that there had been undue emphasis on the sexual difficulties in proportion to time spent on other strains in the relationship. On learning this information, the counselor decided to follow Ms. Robbin's wishes and not discuss sex initially. In this instance, the counselor recognized that sex was a highly sensitive area and it would be better to defer discussion of this issue until Ms. Robbins could take the initiative herself.

Structuring the Interview

Length of Time. Traditionally, a therapeutic session is limited to 45 or 50 minutes, a time block that is usually applied in those cases where the counselor and client are meeting together on a regularly scheduled basis one or more times a week. There may be emergency situations or times of crisis when flexibility is necessary and the client may require more time. When settling on a time that is mutually agreeable, consideration should be given to both the client's and the counselor's interests and schedules. It is not reasonable for a counselor to expect a student to come to his office on a regular basis during school hours, nor is it reasonable to expect a working man to risk losing his job to keep appointments during working hours. On the other hand, it is not reasonable for a client to expect a counselor to give up weekends and every evening to his clients. Therefore, a balance must be reached so that neither the counselor nor the client is inconvenienced.

Setting the Fee. If the counselor is employed by an agency that has a scheduled fee system, then the agency's policies apply. These policies are usually written and quite explicit, showing the income level, the number of family members, and the appropriate fee. It is expected that all beginning clinical interviewers will be working under the auspices of an agency in which the services offered, the hours, and the fees are set down in an agency schedule and are often handled by an administrative person.

If a client inquires about the fee, the counselor should ascertain what prior information the client has received regarding the fee. Some clients who already know the fee and still ask the counselor about it are expressing mistrust of the counselor. They are wondering whether the counselor will give accurate information, whether he is trustworthy, and whether he will answer the client's questions. The counselor should answer the question matter of factly and directly, stating the agency fee that has been established. Later he may take up the issue of the mistrust implied by the question.

Sometimes a client raises questions about the fee because he feels it is too high. The counselor should take the client's objections seriously even if it appears to him that the client can afford the fee. If after discussing the problem the client still feels the fee is unjust, an agreement may be made to review the situation periodically. If the client falls behind in his payments because of limited funds, consideration should be given to setting a lower fee for the client.

If the client has sufficient funds and is not paying because of resistance to counseling, the counselor may try to work on the problem with the client. But if after one or two months the client still refuses to pay, it is wiser to terminate the counseling instead of allowing the situation to drag on. Generally speaking, money is a charged issue both for the counselor and the client and is often of diagnostic significance (see the section on inquiry into embarrassing subjects, Chap. 3).

Ms. Burns, age 35, came into treatment because of depression and concern about her identity as a woman. She worried constantly that she was taking over for her husband and handling his affairs. When the counselor took up the issue of her previous month's unpaid bill, Ms. Burns commented that she did not know of the situation as her husband paid all the bills. This led to a discussion of her conflicts about taking over responsibility for herself in areas other than money. She said that she was afraid of taking responsibility because this represented a masculine role to her. In this case, taking up the issue of the fee reinforced the counseling process by opening up the client's conflict about her femininity.

Mr. Ware, age 28, was referred to treatment by his wife's counselor after Ms. Ware had become psychotic. The appearance of Ms. Ware's symptoms corresponded to her husband's increasing withdrawal of affection and interest in her. Although Mr. Ware had agreed to follow the recommendation, he complained constantly of financial problems and of limited finances. He also felt that his wife was draining him financially, which made him very angry. When Mr. Ware did not pay his first bill, the counselor questioned him as to what the difficulty was. Mr. Ware became angry and told the counselor that he didn't see why he had to come to treatment anyway, and since he really didn't need it, he didn't think he should have to pay. The counselor asked Mr. Ware if he was going to let this minimal fee stand in the way of his dealing with his anger and coping with his disturbed wife. Mr. Ware then admitted that he was certain he could benefit from counseling and agreed to continue. In this case, the counselor postponed specific discussion of the fee in order to make more of an effort to engage the client.

Mr. Golden had come to the agency for counseling because of his compulsiveness in his work and because he frequently took on more responsibilities than he could handle. Although his wife and children were entirely dependent on his salary, he willingly agreed to the established agency fee. When he fell behind in his payments, the counselor was concerned about this unusual behavior and asked the client about it. Mr. Golden explained that he was helping his in-laws with their extra medical expenses and could not make ends meet. He intended to pay his counseling bill in the future. The counselor felt it was advisable to reduce the fee as a way of showing the client that again he had taken on more than he could handle.

Frequency of Contact. Usual clinic practice is for the counselor and client to meet together once a week, with an occasional extra hour as necessary. Some clients can benefit from two or three sessions per week. Whether or not this can be done depends on the counselor's and client's schedules, the client's financial situation, and the regulations of the agency.

The Unwilling Client

It is not always of his own volition that a client comes in for counseling, but because he has been ordered to do so by the court, probation office, or protective services agency or because he or she is the parent of a child in a guidance clinic or is a relative of a hospital patient. It is not unusual for one of these clients to respond to the inquiry of what brought him in by stating, "The judge sent me." The client is thus implying that it is the authority's problem rather than his own. In order for the sessions to be productive, the counselor attempts to turn this attitude around, a task that is usually difficult and sometimes impossible.

The counselor explains his function and the purpose of the interview, and asks the client how this purpose applies to him and what would he like to discuss about it. If his attitude remains negative, the counselor can introduce some general topics that are common to other clients who have been sent by a similar authority. These leads may or may not result in the client's participation. If they fail, the counselor may find it impossible to work with such an unmotivated and resistant client and feel that further discussion would be useless. For example, in a welfare agency, the client may only be interested in obtaining additional funds for her family. She may refuse to discuss anything else until she has received the extra money. The counselor acknowledges that the allowance the client has received is a minimal one and asks how she has been managing so far and what difficulties she has experienced in feeding and clothing the family. The counselor can also bring up other problems such as rent, heat, and overcrowding. The client may or may not respond to the counselor's interest. In some instances, a client will share a problem with the counselor, such as that her husband has returned home unannounced after a six-month disappearance and that she is confused about what to do and what would be best for the children. Another client may insist that her only problem is insufficient funds and refuse to have anything to do with counseling.

> Ms. Sherwood went to a child guidance clinic on the recommendation of her son's teacher. The purpose was to discuss her disturbed, aggressive, and overactive eight-year-old son. During the first interview, the counselor found that Ms. Sherwood was reluctant to return to the clinic as she "did not have any problems" and merely "wanted to straighten her son out." It became apparent to the counselor that Ms. Sherwood did not understand the reasons for involving her in counseling. To elicit Ms. Sherwood's participation in the interview, the counselor asked her to discuss her son's behavior at home and the problems she had noticed. She was encouraged to describe her son's problems in detail. When this had been accomplished, the counselor asked how the boy's behavior had affected the home situation, including the relationships among the family members. In an effort to establish a therapeutic relationship, the counselor attempted to work with the mother to identify problem areas in the home and in that way to break through her denial. If Ms. Sherwood would admit to some problems in the home, it would then be possible to work on them with her.

> Mary, age 15, was sent by the court to a hospital for drug withdrawal and psychiatric treatment. She insisted that all she wanted was methadone and that she had no problems to discuss. Prior efforts with her in psychotherapy had been unsuccessful because she had preferred not to look inside herself. The counselor, in reviewing Mary's prior

therapy as well as Mary's own attempts at self-help, pointed out to her the pattern of repeated failure. The counselor suggested that Mary examine these failures and that they explore together what went wrong. Because Mary was sullen and negative, the counselor had to shift from stressing intrapsychic issues to interpersonal areas that Mary could relate to. The counselor asked her what it was like on the streets and if she had friends there. Mary responded that no one liked her, just as previous counselors had not liked her. This gave the counselor a chance to inquire into the difficulties that prevented people from liking her. Mary was intrigued by the question and tried to find an answer, which was the beginning of a counseling relationship.

Notetaking

Beginning interviewers worry unnecessarily about how they will remember the important features of the interview. If the counselor is giving his full attention to the client, rather than to his notebook, he will find that recalling the important issues under discussion is easily done. The counselor is not expected to remember dates or addresses. He may decide to note these facts for his records and in case he needs to get in touch with the client. If the client asks why full notes are not being taken, the counselor can tell the client that he is giving his attention to the client's reactions and emotions as well as to what he is saying, and notetaking would be a distraction. The counselor can openly admit that he will not remember every detail but will remember general trends and patterns that are indicative of the client's problem and conflicts.

Taking copious notes during a session may prove very distracting to both the client and the counselor. The focus belongs on the client, not on the notebook. It is good practice, however, for the beginner to take 5 or 10 minutes after each interview to write a summary of the relevant issues covered for his own review of the progress of the counseling and for his supervisor.

How to Conclude an Interview

While it is not a good idea to be so rigid as to stop a client in the middle of a sentence, it is important to finish the interview on time. In this way, the client is reminded that there are boundaries to the session as well as to the relationship. Consistency in the counselor's behavior is also important to the client. Beginning and ending an interview on time are a way of showing consistency. Most counselors agree that about 10 minutes before the conclusion of the interview, the counselor should begin to think about the ending of the session. He usually considers further issues that he or the client may wish to bring up and may say to the client, "Our time will be up soon, is there something you would like us to consider further?" or "Have we covered everything you wish to discuss?" It is not necessary for the counselor to give a detailed summary of what has transpired if the sessions are going to be continued. The counselor might comment on specific issues that have been raised and say, "We'll talk more about that next time," or "We ought to go over that some more." This tells the client that there is more work to be done on a particular conflict both inside and outside the office. In initial interviews a client may ask the counselor for an account of how he sees the situation. The counselor makes clear to the client that it is not his place to give an account of the situation, but rather that the client has decisions to make about how he wants to proceed with his life. The client can do what he wants and, especially, what makes sense for him.

It is important that the counselor pace the interview so that adequate time is left for a discussion of plans for future appointments. The client should not have to feel confused or worried about when he will see his counselor again. The counselor can conclude the interview by saying that time is up and indicating the time and date of the next appointment.

For clients who know that they have regular appointments, it is not necessary to repeat the exact date and hour of the next appointment. Instead, the comment "See you next week" is sufficient. It is courteous for the counselor to rise and show the client to the door at the end of the interview.

REFERENCES

1. Schubert M: Interviewing in Social Work Practice: An Introduction. New York, Council on Social Work Education, 1971
2. Sullivan HS: The Psychiatric Interview. New York, Norton, 1954
3. Whitehorn JC: Guide to interviewing and clinical personality study. Arch Neurol and Psychiatry 52:197–216, 1944

5

TYPICAL TECHNICAL PROBLEMS

Various technical problems arise during an interview which may cause difficulties for the beginning counselor. Although the list is not exhaustive, in this chapter we discuss many of the typical problem situations that may crop up occasionally or may occur frequently during the course of the counseling. In practice, problem solving is always carried out with attention to the context in which the problem is being presented and discussed. The following examples present brief descriptions of the therapeutic context of the problems and the techniques used to deal with them.

PROLONGING THE INTERVIEW

Occasionally a client will start a long, detailed story toward the end of an interview. He may be excessively anxious about the interview ending, or he may be unconsciously expressing excessive expectations of the counselor. In either case continuing the interview to allow the client to complete his story is not in the best interests of the client. If the problem is excessive expectation, by extending the time, the counselor feeds the client's fantasy wish for a magical solution. Then when the client does not receive the magical solution, he is disappointed and disillusioned with the counselor. If the problem is extreme anxiety about the session being over, by extending it the counselor is only postponing the end and, in effect, prolonging the client's anxiety, since the session must end eventually. In both cases the client's reasons for attempting to prolong the session must be made conscious and available to open discussion. By prolonging the session, the counselor would be trying to use extra time as a solution rather than facing the issues with the client. Once the counselor understands that staying within the set boundaries is in the client's best interest—and that does not mean cutting the client off in the middle of a sentence or setting an alarm clock—the issue of ending interviews becomes simply another part of counseling to be worked on.

At times like this, when the client keeps talking or appears otherwise reluctant to leave and the counselor's statement "Our time is up" seems to fall on deaf ears, the counselor can ask, "Do you find it hard to leave? If you do, that's something we can talk about next time. It's important that we understand your wish to stay here." This is usually enough to mobilize the client by putting the issue back into a therapeutic context and reducing the element of struggle between client and counselor. Then the client is able to leave with dignity. A stronger measure is for the counselor to stand up and walk to the door. In very rare instances of a special crisis or stress situation that needs further attention, by mutual agreement and plan, the interview may extend beyond the usual time.

CLIENT WANTS TO LEAVE EARLY

Some clients feel so anxious, uncomfortable, or angry that they wish to leave early. This desire may be so overwhelming that they actually begin to leave the office. In most cases it is better for the client to remain and work toward understanding what is pushing him to leave. If he leaves, he might feel embarrassed or guilty or that the counselor is not capable of handling the situation. Accordingly, when a client starts to look uncomfortable or tense, the counselor might inquire in a very matter of fact way about what is making the client so tense or what is so difficult. To a client who worries that the counselor cannot possibly understand him or to an almost uncontrollably anxious client, the counselor says, "I want you to stay and make sense of this." To the client who is less anxious and uncomfortable, he might comment, "It is possible to work on the discomfort so that it becomes understandable and manageable."

There are some clients who mask their anger or anxiety and say they want to leave because they have nothing more to talk about and ask, "What's the use of staying?" The counselor could respond, "You seem to be anxious or angry rather than just bored and even though you feel blocked, how about if we think about it some?" Or he might say, "Running away from feelings is not a solution for anger, but we can talk about it." These are attempts to get the client to look at his reasons for wanting to leave. It is also necessary for the counselor to add in all these situations that there is a difference between wishes and actions, by saying, "Even though you'd like to leave, you don't have to act on it and go; it's possible to understand wishes and how they work without acting on them."

LATENESS

If the client is late repeatedly, it is important to determine to what extent there might be a reality factor (then counselor and client can simply find a better appointment time) or to what extent the lateness represents a means of handling a habitual emotional conflict. When the counselor inquires into the reasons, the client is pushed to look at any resistance or reluctance that might be present and to examine his ambivalence about keeping appointments. The response provides necessary information as to whether the lateness is general or limited to the counseling. If the client says that he is late for everything, then this offers a diagnostic clue as to the nature of the way he relates to people and a comment such as "How come?" may be as far as the counselor can go. It is not appropriate to introduce possibilities such as the client's wish to provoke others or the client's more basic fantasies that he wants to do others damage by keeping them waiting. This can be done when the client can see a pattern in his habitual lateness.

Counseling situations work best when comments are timed to follow the client's capacity to be consciously aware. Often the client will not be aware of what pressure prevents him from arriving on time. The counselor does not press the client to come up with an explanation that is clearly not available to him at that time. In those situations where a client is late only to his counseling appointments, the counselor can begin the discussion of the client's concern about the counseling situation by saying, "We can both keep an eye on it, and by trying to notice what you feel before you get here and after you come, we will begin to get clues as to what is going on." It is only after some evidence about the client's fear of the counseling or perhaps anger at the counselor emerges either directly from the client or indirectly by way of associations that further clarification can occur.

Conversely, if the counselor should happen to be late, the client may feel that he is being rejected or is not very important. Therefore, the counselor apologizes for the delay and makes every effort to be punctual.

CRYING

Crying is a fairly common phenomenon in the therapeutic interview. Sometimes people apologize for crying because they feel embarrassed or worried that it is a sign of weakness. The counselor's response to such apologies may be, "What's wrong with crying?" Ordinarily, it is not advisable to physically comfort an adult client. It is the counselor's choice whether to say nothing or to comment, "What is so disturbing or upsetting that makes you cry?" When the client is recounting a recent or past sad experience such as a loss, crying is predictable, and he can be told this.

There are frequent instances when the causes for crying are unclear to the counselor and to the client. Crying can result from different emotions, such as anger, fear, rage, anxiety, and sadness. Regardless of whether the broad stimulus to crying is clear or unclear, it is useful to ask "What about this makes you cry now?" It is important for diagnostic purposes to distinguish between crying that is caused by global depression and crying that is related to affect-laden situations. For example, a woman cried as she reported that she could not get out of bed in the morning and had no appetite or energy to do anything. This crying differs from that of a man who tearfully related how lonely he felt after his dog was run over and how hard it was to see him buried. The woman's crying revolved around a state of anxiety and depression, whereas the man's crying was due to a loss.

In unusual or exceptional situations, the client's crying can become uncontrollable. At these times the counselor needs to stop the flow of material in an effort to get the client back in control. Don't ask: "Can you pull yourself together?" or "Do you feel you've gone too far?" Instead, the counselor attempts to get the client to understand what he is crying about by such comments as "You seem to feel desperate about the loss of your children (or husband or mother)," or "You seem so lonely and unhappy about your situation." The counselor, by recognizing that the client's loss of control is due to conscious or unconscious problems, tries to get the client to the point of talking rather than crying. Asking a question such as "Do you feel as though this is happening now?" brings the client back to the present reality. When crying seems to stem from unconscious sources, the counselor asks the client if he has any ideas as to the reasons for the crying and offers possible explanations if the crying continues.

There are some situations that seem very sad to the counselor, and the novice may find himself about to cry. If the counselor is unable to control his response, it could endanger the therapeutic relationship. Crying by the counselor would mean overidentification with the client and the loss of emotional neutrality. This loss of control by the counselor makes it difficult for the client to freely express his feelings for fear of upsetting the counselor. Whereas empathy is important in "tuning in" to the client's feelings, overemotionalism is a signal to the counselor to discuss his feelings with his supervisor. If a counselor cries in front of a client, he gives up his professional position of interested, objective neutrality and becomes just like another friend.

SILENCE

Generally, it is not a good idea for the client to remain silent for more than a minute or two. Silence can represent a number of things. It may be related to hostility, withdrawal, resistance, shyness, embarrassment, or blocking, i.e., stopping in the middle of a thought and being unable to go on. Asking the client what he is thinking about will usually interrupt the silence. If the client responds, "Nothing," "I don't know," or is unable to respond, the counselor can handle it in various ways. He can interpret the silence if he has a good idea about its cause. These comments might be related to recent topics under discussion, such as "You seem shy about discussing sex," or "You seem to be experiencing too much pain to continue talking about your mother." If the counselor is uncertain and the client does not respond to his suggestions, the counselor can introduce a new topic or review the previous discussion to enable the client to participate. If the silence persists, a comment such as "I'm not sure what's going on when you're silent and I don't mean to interrupt if it's valuable. Did you feel this way before the session, or is your silence particular to this situation?" If the client does not respond and remains silent, which is unusual, every once in a while indicate that you are still there and are wondering what he is thinking about.

CLIENT UNABLE TO SIT THROUGH THE INTERVIEW

Some clients are so anxious that they cannot remain seated for any length of time and, instead, walk around the office, pace, leave to get water or use the bathroom. Although it would be of more benefit for the client to sit and talk out his anxieties instead of going into action, with some clients the beginner will find it better to accept the client's movements. A counselor does not force a client to sit down. Instead he asks "What is so disturbing that you have to get up from the chair?" Obviously there are many other ways to get the client to look at what he is doing. As long as the counselor keeps in mind that the relationship is that of equals with different tasks, the questions and comments will reflect his efforts to get the client to examine his actions.

Ms. Peterson, age 35, got up and walked around the office whenever she talked about how she might expand her life by developing some interests. As she walked around, she complained that the counselor was putting too much pressure on her and she did not see how she could go to work even though her children were in high school. The counselor pointed out that it was not his pressure, but rather pressure from within that prompted Ms. Peterson's walking around. He suggested that the client sit down and talk about the reason she felt so pressured.

Mr. Redd, age 25, had told his counselor that he was spending most of the day in bed. During his interview whenever the topic of his inactivity and lack of motivation came up, he would rise and leave the room to get a drink or go to the bathroom. When he returned the third time, Mr. Redd commented that he felt criticized and that he could not take it.

PHYSICAL CONTACT

Handshaking on first arrival may be initiated by the client, and if so, the counselor responds as in a first greeting. It is not usual for the client or the counselor to continue this practice beyond the first meeting.

Some clients may want to hold their counselor's hand or touch him in an effort to feel closer to him or to gain impossible ends. If a counselor puts his arm around a client or hugs him, the client may feel threatened by this gesture of closeness and may interpret this as a sexual provocation. An exception is when a client becomes violent and tries to hurt himself. During these very rare times, the counselor will have to physically restrain the client.

Recently, in the popular press, there have been articles describing situations in which psychiatrists have sexual intercourse with their clients. We strongly oppose this practice. Any sexual involvement is unacceptable as it is a reflection of a subjective rather than an objective relationship and precludes further therapeutic work. (See Chap. 2 for a discussion of the boundaries of the therapeutic relationship and the rationale for maintaining a professional stance.)

PERSONAL QUESTIONS

In general, it is unwise for the counselor to offer personal information. However, clients often ask the counselor personal questions. When a client asks a personal question, it is important to understand what the client is concerned about. The client may be asking out of curiosity, out of an attempt to get closer, as a way of experiencing the counselor as a real person, as a manipulation to "become friends," as a way of changing the subject, and so forth.

When the counselor gives personal information too readily, the focus tends to move to the counselor and away from the client, where it should be. When a client asks a question such as "Are you a student?" or "Are you a doctor?" he is usually concerned with the counselor's competence. The counselor, in an effort to get at the client's fears that the counselor is not sufficiently capable of helping him, can respond, "Does it make a difference to you? What is your concern?" If, instead, the counselor readily answers the question, the client may feel that the counselor is weak because he acquiesces to the client's wishes. It is a mistaken "rule," however, that one never gives such information. If the counselor decides to answer, he should be brief and to the point and then return the focus to the client[1(p52)] by saying, "Let us get back to you," or "We were talking about you."

> Ms. Adams, who was a 38-year-old housewife and had two children, was seeing a young counselor and pointedly asked her age. The counselor recognized that the client had doubts about her competence and chose not to give that information but responded, "What is your concern about me?" The client then came out with all her doubts about the counselor, saying, "You are too young, unmarried, and don't have any children, so how can you possibly understand what I am going through?" The counselor acknowledged that she was not married and did not have any children, but she went on to ask how was it that the client, knowing her background and training, would so quickly assume that she was not qualified. By raising the issue in this way, the counselor reassured the client of her competence and at the same time put the issue back into the therapeutic context.

The following analogies or similar ones can be used by the counselor to make it easier for the client to see that a counselor's competence in understanding a certain experience need not be based on his having gone through the same experience. Most obstetricians have never had a baby and yet are able to deliver children. Most surgeons have never experienced operations at which they are expert. And, in the same way, clinicians do not have to experience a problem in order to understand it. More important, the client must recognize that it is his own understanding that is the critical factor.

CANCELLED APPOINTMENTS

There are times when a counselor has to cancel an appointment because he is ill or because of some conflict in his schedule. As soon as the counselor is aware of the need to cancel, he should telephone the client to reschedule the interview. It is permissible to tell the client you are ill or that some conflict in your schedule has come up that necessitates a change. (It is not necessary or even useful to burden the client with detailed personal explanations of the necessary change.) It is unwise to be too vague and say, "I'll be in touch," as this could easily be taken as a rejection or as meaning that you are very sick, or angry or bored. Scheduling a new appointment as close to the original one as possible indicates to the client that you are interested in continuing to work with him. Ambiguity about a new appointment leaves the client uncertain and may give rise to all kinds of fantasies. There is so much ambiguity inherent in the therapeutic situation that it is important to clarify reality factors whenever possible. These same principles apply if a client cancels an appointment. The counselor wants to have as clear an idea as possible whether the cancellation was due to some unavoidable necessity or whether it was the result of an emotional conflict. However, it is often important to find this out subtly and only ask direct questions when it becomes appropriate. Once the counselor thinks that he knows enough about the reason for the cancellation, he will wait to discuss it when he feels it will further the therapeutic work.

CLIENT DOES NOT WANT TO RETURN

There may be times when the client does not want to return and refuses to make another appointment. When this happens, the counselor asks the client what his reasons are for not wanting to return and discusses them with him. The client might admit that he had been angry with the counselor and had felt that they could no longer work together. This kind of reaction, as well as other misunderstandings, needs to be cleared up.

> Ms. Brown, age 40, began an interview by stating that she was not going to continue the counseling. Her family had to move, and she needed the time to look for a new apartment. Besides, she felt angry about a statement that the counselor had made at the conclusion of the last interview. The counselor had recommended joint therapy for her and her husband, and she felt she was being pushed aside. Ms. Brown said she did not agree with the counselor's view that she and her husband were not communicating, and this had led her to feel that the counselor did not understand her. After admitting and discussing her feelings of rejection, Ms. Brown made another appointment.

Some clients telephone to cancel an appointment and either do not make another one or do not show up the next time. In these instances, the counselor telephones to inquire about the client and to offer him another appointment. If a client repeats this behavior and it becomes a pattern, the counselor might consider phoning or writing to clarify the status of the counseling. There may be times when the counselor is truly worried about a client who has not kept an appointment because of the possibility of serious harm to himself or others. During these exceptional times, it may be necessary to visit the client at his home or to ask the police to do so.

It is not unusual for a beginning counselor to come up against a client who does not want to return or who insists on seeing someone else. The client may have hoped for a counselor who was older, of a different sex, or perhaps was still hoping to find someone with the answers. It is not in the client's best interest for the counselor to coerce him to return by threatening a bleak future. It is equally inappropriate to seduce the client by promising a cure or the answer to his problems. Sometimes even the best efforts at exploring the refusal to return fail. Then the counselor must remember that it is not possible to force the client's further participation, and he must accept his own limitations and those of the client.

EXTRA APPOINTMENTS

When a client is in the midst of a crisis or is especially upset during an interview and it seems that the upset is not abating, the counselor may suggest an extra appointment. In this way, the counselor acknowledges his interest in a client who is unusually disturbed.

> After losing his job, Mr. Budd, age 40, had become quite depressed and despondent, was staying at home, was rarely socializing, and seemed generally immobile. When he was offered a job several hundred miles away, he became extremely agitated and confused about what decision to make. He was torn between his local ties, especially to his sick mother and to a city that he loved, and economic security in a rural section of the country. Because he seemed in so much turmoil, the counselor suggested that an extra appointment might be useful at this time. In this instance, the client might have suggested the appointment himself, but because he felt so undeserving he was unable to ask for special consideration.

When the client does ask for an extra appointment, it is important to explore the motivation behind the request. The client may have a genuine need for extra time, or he may be testing the counselor to see if he cares about him or to see how permissive he is. Regardless of the counselor's decision or whether or not the issues are clear, the counselor must be ready to explain to the client how he reached the decision he made. The following examples demonstrate the difference between clients who can use additional appointments and those for whom the request itself is an issue for discussion.

> Mr. Burns, age 35, a very suspicious man who personalized every situation, asked for an extra appointment when there was a reorganization at work. Some of his colleagues were being fired, and he was worried that he too was going to lose his job. He wanted an extra appointment in order to sort out what was reality and what were irrational worries on his part. During this crisis situation, the counselor agreed that Mr. Burns was finding it difficult to handle himself at work and recognized the possibility of his behavior getting out of hand, thus jeopardizing his job. Both Mr. Burns and the counselor understood that it would be useful to have more time to discuss these issues.

> Ms. Price, age 30, was referred for counseling because she had become very depressed and had begun to think about suicide when her mother died. She reported that throughout her life she had longed for a close relationship with her mother but had always felt unwanted and a burden. Although she wanted to make new relationships, she was afraid to do so. When she requested an extra appointment, the counselor asked for her reasons for the request. Ms. Price berated the counselor for not caring or understanding and for being "just like her mother." In

this instance, the counselor explained to Ms. Price that an extra appointment might represent to her a fulfillment of her wish that the counselor take her mother's place. Instead, the counselor suggested that the client work toward a better understanding of her relationship with her mother and her wishes for a replacement.

SMOKING

It is preferable that neither the counselor nor the client smoke during the interview as it is distracting and may interfere with the process of the interview. Nonetheless, many clients still smoke, and a client may ask the counselor for a cigarette or matches. If this only happens once, the counselor may not want to take it up as an issue. But if it occurs repeatedly, the counselor and the client should probably examine the client's behavior, which may be indicative of a dependency conflict.

> Mr. Dodd, age 23, lived at home with his mother and was unemployed. He entered treatment in an effort to break away from his mother and to get a job. After several appointments, in which he requested matches, the counselor asked him how was it that he did not carry his own. At first Mr. Dodd answered, "Either I forget to carry them, or I just lose them." The counselor looked unconvinced by this answer. This led Mr. Dodd to say, "I guess I have trouble looking after myself."

Sometimes the client will offer a counselor a cigarette. Whether or not the counselor smokes, the best way to handle this is to simply say, "No, thank you." Any action by the counselor of offering or accepting cigarettes may be given special meaning by the client.

CONFIDENTIALITY

Verbal confidentiality means that subjects under discussion will not be mentioned by the counselor outside of this professional relationship or without the client's permission. Usually, the client and the counselor come to a mutual agreement about what information can be transmitted. For the most part confidentiality does not come up as an issue as the client assumes the counselor is a responsible, professional person whom he can trust. He knows that his personal information will only be shared with selected professionals with his permission, but he may not always know when or if this takes place. Indeed, it is inappropriate for a counselor to discuss cases in the corridors, to mention case anecdotes in social settings, or to read case records in public view. Similarly, if the client asks about other clients, it is reassuring to the client to learn that the material is held in confidence and not shared with him or anyone else.

If honest, factual statements about the ethics of confidentiality do not satisfy the client and he continues to worry, then it is obvious his worry is an indication of an underlying concern such as a family secret, inability to trust anyone, and so forth. Further exploration into the roots of the client's worries are undertaken in the context of the therapeutic process, not for the defense of the ethics of the relationship.

> Mr. North, age 45, was seeking marital counseling as he had become involved with another woman but was still very tied to his wife and children. He was reluctant to go into details about his relationship with the new woman because he was worried that the counselor would reveal the situation to his wife. It is in reality the client's task to decide whether or not he wants to openly acknowledge his other relationship. His lack of trust in the counselor indicates his own doubts as to whether he can trust himself. A reply such as "What makes you think I will tell your wife?" forces the client to look at this.

RECORD KEEPING

Record keeping by the counselor is usually taken for granted, and clients rarely mention it. But there are a few who ask to see their records. The counselor usually refuses these requests by quoting agency policy. There are some clients who do not ask to see the record directly, but do want to know what is in it. Every client understands the importance of noting identifying data and some general summary statements. If the client seems overly concerned or preoccupied with his record, exploring these worries may yield an assessment of the degree of his suspiciousness or lack of trust. The client's concern over his record may be due to his possible involvement in a court action, such as divorce, guardianship, court hearings regarding an arrest, or hospital commitment. When there is potential for legal complications, it is important that the record be factual and nonjudgmental. With such complicated matters, agency policy and conferences with supervisors offer the most direct guidance about the method for proceeding.

The main purpose of keeping records is for agency accountability to the client, and it is therefore the client's interest that is paramount when the counselor dictates or writes in the record. Personal informal notes kept by the counselor as reminders (see the section Notetaking, Chap. 4) are kept in a locked file or destroyed when they are no longer needed. In Chapter 9, record keeping is discussed as a means for supervision.

Agencies have strict policies about releasing information to requesting agents, and, again, clients can be told of agency policies. In fact, if a client wants or agrees to have his record sent out, he is required to sign a written statement authorizing this. Client and counselor together discuss what is to be included. When there are court proceedings, a record may be subpoenaed; this is handled by the administration department of the agency or institution in which the counselor works.

TRUTHFULNESS

A counselor should not lie or distort information that he passes on to a client. If he is concerned about the client's reaction to some disturbing news or information, it is better to tell the truth. The need for the counselor to give the client such information often occurs in relation to death, divorce, catastrophic illness, or accident. If the client asks directly about a specific reality situation, the counselor acknowledges the facts that he knows and goes on to deal with the client's reactions.

In interdisciplinary settings, such as a hospital or child guidance clinic where more than one member of the family is involved in treatment, this matter is dealt with by an agreement between the family member and the counselor as to who says what to the original client, and when. The most propitious time to initiate the discussion depends on the condition of the client.

Ms. Quinn, age 30, had a very close relationship with her father, who was living with Ms. Quinn's sister in another state. Ms. Quinn was living in an apartment and having difficulty keeping a job. She was in treatment to find out her reasons for "sabotaging" herself. When her father died, her sister telephoned the counselor and requested that he tell the client of her father's death because she was afraid of how her sister would react to the news. The counselor agreed with the sister that it was important that the client be told the news in a setting in which there would be someone with whom she could discuss her feelings. He preferred that the sister and Ms. Quinn handle the loss together, but the sister was too upset and fearful about her sister's vulnerability to break the news to her in a long-distance telephone call. When Ms. Quinn arrived for her appointment, the counselor told her that he had some sad news for her and explained that her sister had called regarding her father's death. The client was quite startled by the news and asked why her sister had not told her directly. This led to further discussion about the repetitive family pattern of infantilizing the client, assuming her to be weak and vulnerable. The client recognized the undesirability of the counselor's assuming this family role as it played into her sister's, as well as her own, poor picture of herself. The counselor's frank relating of the news to Ms. Quinn, including the sister's feelings, led to a discussion in which the client learned something about herself, and thus profited from the situation.

The counselor should not overlook misconceptions on the part of the client that have to do with his view of the counselor. If overlooked, these misconceptions, when discovered, give rise to a lack of trust in the counselor. For example, a client may address a single, female counselor with neither an M.D. nor a Ph.D. degree as "Mrs. Jones" or "Dr. Smith." It would be a mistake for the counselor to let the matter go on the assumption that the client might feel better being in treatment with someone who is married or who has more professional status. Later, when the client learned the truth, he would be justified in feeling deceived by the counselor. A "slip" due to misinformation on the part of the client is easily corrected by the counselor simply stating the truth. When the slip is repetitive, it is therapeutic to point out the mistake and inquire into it. This gives the client an opportunity to express his feelings about the counselor, including any doubts he may have. In this instance, the sharing of personal information is necessary to clarify a distortion. This situation is the opposite of the one in which the client asks the counselor if he is a student in an effort to put him in a weak or unqualified position. However, they are similar in that the client is expressing an emotional need or conflict in both. In both situations, clarification of any ambiguity and exploration into the client's doubts are necessary.

TELEPHONE CALLS DURING THE DAY

Counselors often receive telephone calls during the day, either during interviews or in between. Sometimes the call is suggested by the counselor who feels the client may need some support in addition to his regular appointment. The client deserves the counselor's courtesy of listening to what is on his mind. By listening long enough and carefully, the counselor can usually determine if the matter can wait until the next interview or if a longer telephone conversation is in order. If the counselor is busy or in session, he may want to arrange to talk later when it would be more convenient. In a rare emergency situation, the counselor drops everything else and attends to the emergency.

Generally speaking, phone calls during appointments are to be avoided as they are distracting to both the client and the counselor and may cause the client to feel rejected or unimportant. It may be necessary on occasion to accept a phone call in response to a special problem. We do not agree with the view that stresses the usefulness of accepting phone calls during appointments to show the client that there are other reality situations that require the counselor's attention.[2(p 437)] We do agree with letting the client know about reality factors whenever possible, but as there are so many opportunities for this within the therapeutic context, they do not need to be intruded into the situation. Thus, we feel that if the counselor is receiving more than one call during a session, the client's annoyance may be justified, and, therefore, phone calls are to be kept at a minimum.

> Ms. Dole, age 40, was quite preoccupied with her husband's depression and her son's behavior problems as she felt responsible for both. She phoned her counselor constantly to report day-to-day incidents that had occurred between herself and the members of her family, without differentiating their importance or critical significance. The counselor, whose sessions were being interrupted so frequently, suggested to Ms. Dole that they work out some ground rules for these telephone calls and work toward the client's understanding of her need to make the calls. He did not forbid Ms. Dole to telephone, but he did ask her the reasons for the calls. As a result, Ms. Dole began to examine her lack of confidence in herself and her need to rely on others.

EMERGENCIES

The most difficult aspect of an emergency is determining whether the situation is truly an emergency or whether the client involved is so overly anxious or excited that he is responding as if he were in a state of crisis. The counselor's first task is to assess with the client whether the situation calls for such an acute reaction or whether the client's response is excessive and determined by old reaction patterns. A detailed description of the problem or situation by the client clarifies or puts into perspective the extent of the emergency and the client's reaction to it. If the client and counselor determine together that the situation is indeed an emergency, immediate action is warranted.

If at all possible the client takes action in his own behalf even though he may require some direction from the counselor to do so. There may be times when the counselor realizes that the client is either immobilized or so impelled toward self-destruction that the counselor must step in and take action himself.

Jane, age 15, and on drugs, was brought to a walk-in center by her boyfriend, Brad, who had become concerned when she became groggy and sleepy. He was quite frightened and worried that she had taken too many drugs. Whereas Brad wanted to unburden himself to the counselor regarding his guilt about having introduced Jane to drugs, the counselor felt that Jane needed immediate medical attention, and therefore he called a police ambulance. Brad was fearful about Jane's going to the hospital, as he had hoped such a drastic step would not be necessary. It was the counselor's support that induced Brad to accompany Jane to the hospital. In this way Brad could be of further help to Jane by demonstrating his interest and concern. Also, his own excessive guilt feelings would be lessened by his participation in getting proper care for her.

Ms. Porter, age 38, was seeing a counselor because of long-standing marital problems. Her husband was an angry man who often demeaned and insulted her. This contributed to her own self-doubts and caused her frequent agitation. One day Ms. Porter called her counselor crying uncontrollably that she was "falling apart" because her husband had threatened to leave her that very morning. She demanded that the counselor see her husband immediately and stop him from taking such action. Ms. Porter's hysteria seemed out of proportion to the situation as Mr. Porter had frequently told her he was going to leave her. The counselor asked Ms. Porter to describe the morning's events. She told him of her husband's becoming angry after she had failed to get up and prepare his breakfast. Mr. Porter began to yell that either she shape up or he would take off. Because of her highly agitated state, Ms. Porter had taken this to be a final ultimatum on her husband's part. The counselor reminded her that this was not a new threat and that on several other occasions her husband had become so angry that he had also threatened to leave. Instead of agreeing to see Mr. Porter, the counselor pointed out to Ms. Porter that her pattern of overreacting needed further understanding and work. Thus, the client's situation was not considered to be an emergency but a part of the ongoing therapeutic work.

CRISIS INTERVENTION*

Good counseling can be short- or long-term. Frequently a crisis precipitates a client's seeking out a counselor. At such a moment direct intervention on the part of the counselor can head off serious difficulties. At such times counselors need to intervene and then get out—thus permitting the capacities of the individuals involved, which were temporarily disrupted by the crisis or stress, to regain their full working ability.

However, it is equally important to distinguish the genuine acute crisis that has disrupted an ordinarily well integrated person or situation from a chronic chaotic life style in which there is a new crisis much of the time. In the latter case, brief intervention is not particularly useful. In fact, the client who has attempted to get into counseling and has a reasonable expectation that the counselor will understand the chronicity becomes more disappointed and bewildered after a brief intervention.

A crisis occurs as a result of a stressful or hazardous event that disrupts a person's usual equilibrium.[3 (p 24)] This stress may be caused by a separation or a loss. Other sources of tension include an acute or chronic illness, a change in the family situation, or a change from one developmental stage to another. Occurrences such as marriages, divorces, births, deaths, school departures, changes of economic status, moving, and so on, can be so stressful

*We are particularly indebted to Gerald Caplan, M.D., Lydia Rapoport, and Howard J. Parad, whose formulations constitute the basis of this section.

as to create a crisis state. Obviously, many people handle such crisis experiences appropriately, but many others become acutely concerned because the issue has some unusual personal relevance for them.

The characteristics of people in crisis include high anxiety, tension, guilt, depression, anger, withdrawal, lack of appetite, restlessness, and confusion about what is happening. When a client is overreacting to a crisis situation, early intervention is indicated.

Crisis work includes keeping explicit focus on the crisis through:

1. Conscious understanding by the client of the struggle for cognitive mastery. This is accomplished by identifying the problem through techniques of:
   a. exploration and clarification,
   b. working through the individual's doubts about himself,
   c. working through the individual's anticipatory worries and offering guidance for coping.
2. Offering basic information and education.
3. Finding a bridge to community resources by bringing in other family members or friends, or contacting the appropriate agency. In this type of work, the counselor is active and offers the client a sense of hope and mastery in the crisis. The counselor must be more accessible and more to the point in a crisis situation than in regular therapy. The counselor shares his perceptions of the problem with the client, thus enabling the client to:
   a. get a manageable understanding of the situation,
   b. lower his anxiety,
   c. develop trust in the counselor's competency,
   d. feel understood,
   e. feel a sense of hope of improvement.[4] (p 56)

John, age 16, came to the school counselor at the suggestion of his teacher who had noticed that he had withdrawn from his peers and had been crying in the restroom. Until that day, John had been a leader of his group, an excellent student, cheerful, and very responsive to others. Because the teacher felt that such a drastic change in his behavior required special attention, he referred John to the school counselor. In talking with John about what was wrong, the counselor learned that the boy's father had been in an automobile accident the night before and had been seriously injured. His mother had insisted he go to school, and she went to the hospital.

John told the counselor how attached he was to his father and how worried he was that his father might die. John was an only child, and he and his father had been great buddies. His mother had not told him in detail about his father's condition and insisted he go to school and carry on his usual routines. He was unable to study or concentrate in school because he was so worried about his father. The counselor realized that John needed more information about his father's condition and the opportunity to be with him. The counselor telephoned John's mother to let her know he was planning to send John to the hospital. She was relieved to hear from the counselor as she had been torn between sending John to school and taking him with her. In fact, she preferred to pick him up so that he would not have to make the trip alone. John was grateful for the counselor's understanding and immediate response to his acute distress.

REFERENCES

1. Garrett A: Interviewing: Its Principles and Methods, 2nd ed. New York, Family Service Association of America, 1972
2. MacKinnon RA, Michels R: The Psychiatric Interview in Clinical Practice. Philadelphia, Saunders, 1971
3. Parad HJ (ed): Crisis Intervention: Selected Readings. New York, Family Service Association of America, 1965
4. Rapoport L: Working with families in crisis: an exploration in preventive intervention. Soc Work 7(1):48–56, 1962

6

THE UNPREDICTABLE

In the course of clinical practice there will always be unplanned events and special issues that require quick thought and flexibility on the part of the counselor if they are to be dealt with in a way that will be therapeutic for the client and not merely disruptive. Simply knowing about such possibilities offers the counselor some preparation. The following are some examples of unplanned events and the techniques used to help incorporate the unpredictable into a therapeutic context.

AN UNEXPECTED ARRIVAL

There may be times when the client will arrive in the company of a relative or friend, with the expectation of including this person in the interview. Before the client enters the office, the counselor usually inquires about the reason for the presence of the other person. This interaction with the client enables the counselor to learn what may have precipitated this unusual procedure.

Because bringing in another person may be a positive step or it may be a form of resistance, the motivation can only be evaluated in terms of that particular individual. Usually the client can be seen alone before the counselor decides whether or not to include the visitor. Sometimes after this brief discussion the counselor is unsure about including the visitor and would prefer not to but realizes that the client feels strongly about the matter. Under those circumstances it is probably wiser to acknowledge the client's wishes and accede to the request, at least initially. As the interview progresses the counselor along with the client and the visitor can decide about continuing.

Occasionally a husband will bring his wife to the appointment or vice versa. A counselor might refuse to see the spouse if a client had been insisting he wanted the counselor to "straighten the wife out" and get her to stop running around. On the other hand, a counselor might be very willing to have a conjoint interview if the husband had been concerned about his wife's withdrawing from him and had persuaded her to come in to talk things over.

Ms. Graham, 33 years old and divorced, was referred for assistance in finding suitable living arrangements apart from her paternal aunt and uncle with whom she was currently living. In addition, it was hoped that she could be motivated to seek employment as she had been unemployed for many years due to her suspiciousness of others and feelings of inferiority. On her first appointment Ms. Graham arrived accompanied by her aunt, who had not planned to participate in the interview. The client invited her aunt in, stating that she did not want to have any secrets from her aunt and wanted her to hear everything that was said. Since this was the initial interview, with the goals of the counseling being to encourage independence and more self-assurance, the counselor decided to see the client alone first. She told the client that she thought they should get acquainted before including her aunt and that the aunt could join them at a later point in the session or at another time.

Bob, age 16, had a long history of taking drugs. He kept his appointments quite regularly, but he was not going to school and often stayed away from home overnight. During the two months of treatment Bob had not yet made a commitment to giving up drugs and did not yet feel that he could trust the counselor. On one occasion he brought a friend along, and they were both most persistent about having a joint interview. When Bob was asked the reason for wanting his friend to participate, he could not give a concrete explanation and just said the two of them did everything together. Because the counselor was still struggling to understand this client, he decided they might learn more by going along with the request and saw the two boys together.

TELEPHONE CALLS AT HOME

Because most beginners work in clinics, hospitals, or walk-in centers, which usually offer coverage for emergencies, counselors need not give out their home telephone numbers when clients ask for them. The agency screens calls, and the counselor is contacted only when the agency considers it to be necessary. Some agency policies explicitly forbid counselors to give out their home telephone numbers.

Other agencies leave the decision of giving out home numbers to the counselor. There are clients who, because they are very disturbed or are in a desperate situation, benefit from knowing their counselor's home telephone number. This extra support enables these clients to feel more secure and, thus, to function better between appointments. It is well to set some ground rules as to the use of the number. For example, a counselor might prefer to be called between 8 P.M. and 10 P.M. during the week or after 10 A.M. on weekends and only if there is a genuine reason. A counselor can find the interviewing excessively onerous if he is subject to continual demands and interruptions by his clients. Setting limits protects the counseling. Also, it is important that the client's wish to phone the counselor be taken up as a therapeutic issue.

Some clients may manage to obtain the counselor's telephone number without his knowing it and call unexpectedly. Under these circumstances, the counselor should be courteous, listen to what the client is saying, and determine if the matter can wait until the next interview. If it cannot wait, it should be dealt with as briefly as possible. A beginning counselor may not be able to handle an emergency completely, and thus in most settings the supervisor or a person on call is available for assistance.

Ms. Barns, age 23, began treatment because she had become excessively concerned that her co-workers were against her. She led a sheltered life and still resided with her parents. When they went on vacation and she was left alone, she became frightened that someone would break into the house and hurt her. One evening her fears became intolerable to her, and she obtained the counselor's phone number and called him. She told the counselor that she was terrified of staying alone and wanted some help in arranging another living situation as soon as possible. Her fears were so overwhelming that she could not think of alternatives on her own. In this case, the counselor was able to point out that although Ms. Barns was terribly frightened, she had been managing for some time. They went over the work they had done in the counseling through which Ms. Barns had recognized how irrational her fears were. They agreed that matters could hold until their next appointment two days later.

The next night Ms. Barns called again. This time they not only went over the same things, but Ms. Barns commented on how reassuring it was to her to have the counselor's telephone number. This gave the counselor the opportunity to point out that the task was not just to reassure her and set up another situation very much like the one with her parents but to work out these excessive fears. This last interaction was gone over in the appointment the next day. A week later there was another phone call in which they went over the same material as in the last one. Gradually Ms. Barns recognized that it was not to her advantage to simply shift her dependency from her parents to the counselor.

Ms. Rogers, age 30, felt entitled to constant attention from everyone including her counselor. In the early stages of counseling Ms. Rogers began to call the counselor whenever she had a disagreement with her boyfriend or her mother. She wanted to talk things over as the incidents were occurring and felt a sense of urgency about calling. Because the counselor felt inundated by unnecessary calls, he told Ms. Rogers over the phone that the problems did not seem to be emergencies and could wait for discussion until their next interview. When the counselor next saw Ms. Rogers, he explained that she would have to learn to tolerate delay as she could not expect people to meet her wishes immediately. The counselor also suggested that they work toward understanding Ms. Rogers' sense of urgency at those times so that she could learn to control this feeling instead of having to act on it.

GIFTS

There may be various reasons for a client to offer his counselor a gift. The client's motivation needs to be understood in order for the counselor to determine whether or not to accept the gift. If the gift is an attempt to personalize the relationship, by making a special friend or parent of the counselor, it is not appropriate to accept the gift. In refusing the gift, the counselor can explain the refusal in the context of the therapeutic relationship. If he prefers, the counselor can simply state that it is agency policy not to accept personal gifts. If the client is persistent, he can be referred to the director of the agency who takes care of such matters.

In some settings, it is quite usual to give candy or some token gift at Christmastime, and these may be graciously accepted with a brief "Thank you." The counselor may prefer to open the gift in front of the client to be sure it is both inexpensive and appropriate. Some clients are very artistic and creative and may present the counselor with one of their own creations. The counselor decides to accept it or return it depending on the issues in the treatment relationship.

> At Christmastime a couple who were in treatment together brought the counselor a plant for the office. They stated that they bought it because they appreciated the interest the counselor had consistently shown them. The counselor felt the gift was appropriate, accepted it, and thanked them.

> A counselor refused a gift as inappropriate to their situation when a client brought her jewelry that he had inherited from his mother as he felt he had no one else with whom to share it. The counselor pointed out to the client that the jewelry had a very personal and special meaning to him, and, therefore, she could not accept it.

> A 30-year-old housewife brought her counselor a scarf, which she had purchased while on vacation. The client made it clear that she was bringing scarves to all her friends as small tokens of her affection. The counselor refused the gift, commenting that it was comparable to the client's previous dinner invitations and pointing out that the gift would not be appropriate within the context of their relationship as it might interfere with their chances of working out her wish to include him among her usual friends.

Ordinarily a counselor does not give gifts to adult clients. An exception might be made if a client with whom he had worked over a period of time graduated from college and the counselor wanted to send a neutral gift such as a book or a record. There are many occasions, such as a wedding or special anniversary, when a card or personal note is very much in order. When working with adolescents, it is usual for the counselor to send a birthday card or give a gift to acknowledge the occasion.[1] (p 15)

SHARING A RIDE

If the counselor is planning to accompany his client to a job interview, family-care home, school admission interview, shopping trip, and so on, the counselor drives the client in his car or the agency car. Adult clients in contrast to adolescents do not usually offer to drive their counselors home nor request a ride home for themselves because it complicates the professional relationship. There may be occasional exceptions, such as snowstorms, bus strikes, subway tie-ups, or physical illness, when the counselor may want to offer or accept a ride. Adolescents require much more flexibility, and taking the client for a ride might be part of the therapeutic process.

COMPLIMENTS

The counselor is faced with the choice of accepting compliments without further examination and merely saying thank you, or smiling, or taking the route of further exploration.

> A young man was in treatment with an attractive female counselor. In an effort to be flirtatious, seductive, and masculine, he frequently began his interviews with a compliment about how pretty the counselor's eyes were or how attractive her dress was. The counselor found it easier to ignore these comments than to question their place in this professional situation. Such questions might hurt the client's feelings. However, she was careful to make sure she was not encouraging these remarks.

If a pattern of frequent compliments emerges, it needs to be discussed. The counselor might want to ask the client what such remarks are all about.

> Ms. Shore, age 50, frequently complimented the counselor on her attractiveness as well as her capabilities. She also would thank the counselor after each interview for listening to her problems. The counselor felt that Ms. Shore was attempting to be ingratiating to her just as she was to others and asked her to look into this behavior. Ms. Shore then was able to report that she felt people did not care about her and, therefore, she tried to win them over with compliments.

It is unusual for a counselor to compliment a client on his appearance or behavior unless there is a specific therapeutic purpose to be accomplished. For example, if a client who is usually very dishevelled or unkempt in appearance arrives looking neat and orderly, the counselor may want to comment that he is glad to see the client "put together" today and inquire into the change. The situation might be reversed with an overly meticulous client. Usual types of social compliments, such as "That's a good-looking coat," are better left out of the counselor-client relationship.

INVITATIONS

Clients will sometimes invite their counselor to a wedding, anniversary, bar mitzvah, engagement luncheon, graduation, testimonial, or other special occasion in their lives. Depending on the nature of the relationship and the goals of counseling, the counselor may or may not elect to attend the celebration. Before accepting an invitation, the client and counselor discuss the meaning of the counselor's attendance as well as how the client plans to introduce the counselor to family and friends. This is necessary because the counselor, if questioned, would have to tell the truth as to who he is. In all likelihood people would know of the counselor's presence, and the client needs to agree to and understand this before going ahead with the invitation.

There are many contraindications to attendance at such events. If the client has not shared with his friends and relatives the fact that he is in treatment and would feel embarrassed if they found out, it would not be wise for the counselor to accept the client's invitation. The issue is probably of greater importance in situations where the client plans to remain in treatment or may want to return at some future time. In these cases the client may want the counselor to participate in the event in order to feel that the counselor is more subjectively involved and has given up the objectivity of the therapeutic relationship. This wish to include the counselor in the "family" rarely can be worked through so that the counselor can join in. More often it cannot be worked on sufficiently in advance or, even if it is, both client and counselor can then see that the attendance at the event is not worth the risk to their relationship.

A client just starting treatment usually does not invite the counselor to a social occasion. When such invitations are forthcoming early, they are generally easy to refuse. Problems about invitations are more likely to occur in the course of long-term counseling where an intense relationship has been established.

It is very unusual for a client to invite his therapist for a drink, lunch, dinner, movies, and so forth, except when he is trying to personalize the relationship or be seductive and flirtatious. It is easier for a beginner to refuse this kind of invitation by simply stating, "No, thank you, it's not possible." If the client's flirtatious behavior persists, the counselor needs to examine his own behavior as to its provocativeness. More experienced counselors usually inquire about the meaning of an invitation with a comment such as "What is it all about?" Inquiry of this nature is more profitable for the client as it leads to a better understanding of what he is looking for in his relationship with the counselor.

As the following examples illustrate, exploration at every level, including fantasies and unconscious yearnings, are necessary before a decision about accepting an invitation is made.

> Susan had entered therapy at 15 because of impulsive behavior, thoughts of suicide, obesity, and trouble coping with her older sister's emotional illness. Through counseling she had shown much improvement, had finished high school, and had entered college. There she found her first boyfriend and quickly became engaged. Although the counselor questioned the advisability of the forthcoming marriage, as Susan was still quite immature and unprepared to handle such responsibility, Susan insisted on going ahead with her plans. When she invited the counselor to the wedding, the counselor accepted. She felt that it was important to attend the ceremony. This would show Susan that the counselor was still available to her and might make it easier for Susan to continue treatment after her marriage. The reasons for accepting as well as how to introduce the counselor were discussed. By the time of the event, Susan was prepared to handle this in a reasonably natural way.

> Mr. Cole, a 28-year-old architect, was in therapy because of depression and inability to function at work. As he began to improve, he became productive at work and won an award for one of his designs. The award was being presented at a dinner in his honor, and he invited the

counselor to attend. In discussing the reasons for the invitation, the client stated that since his father was dead, he would like the counselor to be there in his place. The counselor refused because he felt that it would not be in the client's best interest. He explained to the client that he had to further work through his feelings about his father's death, and the counselor's attendance would serve to foster the client's unrealistic fantasies regarding his feelings about his counselor taking his father's place.

BIRTHS, SERIOUS ILLNESSES, AND DEATHS

At the time of births, serious illnesses, or deaths, the counselor may want to acknowledge the event and does so by sending a card or personal note, whichever he prefers. In the case of a death, it is preferable to send a condolence letter rather than a commercial card as it is thoughtful to show more personal concern at this time. A personal note can serve to foster the client's awareness of his grief and prepare the ground for further work in this area, especially if he is unable to keep appointments during this crisis.

In the event of a death in the client's family, the counselor may decide to attend a wake or funeral, or to pay a condolence call.

> Ms. Croft's father died during the course of treatment. In discussing the funeral arrangements with the counselor, Ms. Croft made it clear that the counselor's presence at the church service would provide the extra support she needed to carry her through. The counselor did attend as he also felt that such support was indeed necessary.

When a client is physically ill and requires hospitalization, a visit to the hospital may be considered. If the hospitalization is planned, the client and counselor can discuss in advance the advisability of the counselor's visiting in the hospital, and they are usually able to avoid visits that would complicate the therapeutic process. In most cases if a client is sick enough to require hospitalization, his physical condition is usually a deterrent to counseling because of his preoccupation with his medical problems. However, there are some clients who have such low self-esteem that a visit during hospitalization can be supportive and demonstrative of the counselor's concern. A brief visit to show continued interest and concern may be all that is necessary.

Sometimes physical illness, particularly with hospitalization, can precipitate severe anxiety. The counselor may be called by the client or the attending physician to see if work with the client could be useful to prevent or eliminate severe anxiety, which might distort a diagnosis or interfere with the medical treatment. Before stepping in, the counselor makes sure that the client and his physician are clear and in agreement about the counselor's participation. Above all, he does not want to complicate the medical problems by causing a conflict with the proper hospital regimen. Once the way is clear, the counselor may find that the illness has exacerbated problems that he and the client were already discussing. When the client can see his anxieties in this larger framework and recognize that his current response does not derive from the present painful situation, he often relaxes.

> Mr. Ladd, age 35, had undergone an emergency hernia operation. Because the hospitalization was unplanned and Mr. Ladd had few contacts with relatives or friends, the counselor felt it was important to pay him a visit to show his interest. The client could not do any therapeutic work from his sickbed and instead regaled the counselor with the details of his operation. Subsequently, he told the counselor how important the visit was to him. The client felt that the visit proved that his fears of abandonment were unrealistic.

> Mr. English, age 40, was scheduled to have an operation on his back that would require two to three weeks of hospitalization. The client was able to talk about his wish that his parents, who lived in a distant city, visit him. The counselor asked if the client wished that he too visit him. The client admitted his wish that the counselor visit him but said he knew that this was childish and that it would be better to wait until he was out of the hospital and could keep his next office appointment.

INFORMAL MEETING OUTSIDE THE OFFICE

Occasionally the counselor and the client may run into each other outside the office, such as in a store, restaurant, or on the street. If the counselor and client are by themselves, it is customary to say hello, but it is not necessary to stop and have a conversation. If the client is uncomfortable in seeing the counselor, he may prefer to avoid a face-to-face meeting. The counselor takes the cue from the client's actions. If the client or counselor is with someone else, it is easier not to get involved with introductions, and again a limited greeting is appropriate. When the client has ignored the counselor, although it is obvious that he was seen, the counselor takes this up in the next session. He might ask the client what his reactions were regarding the encounter, in an effort to bring the client's feelings into the discussion.

> Ms. Greenwood, age 45, was in treatment because of depression and difficulty coping with her daughter's emotional illness. She was with her daughter when she saw the counselor and the counselor's wife at a local restaurant. As Ms. Greenwood walked by the counselor, she smiled and continued toward her table. The counselor likewise acknowledged the client with a smile and also walked on. During the next appointment Ms. Greenwood mentioned the meeting at the restaurant, stating that she did not stop to chat as she knew it was not the thing to do. She thanked the counselor for just smiling because she would have felt embarrassed in front of her daughter had she stopped to talk. The client did not ask, nor did the counselor volunteer, the identity of the woman with him.

SPECIAL REQUESTS

A client may ask his counselor to see a friend, relative, or other person who is in need of treatment. The counselor may elect to see this person for consultation and referral or may choose to refer him elsewhere rather than get involved himself. Generally speaking, a referral to a colleague is simpler and less likely to create problems.

> Mr. Powers, a 20-year-old college student, asked his counselor if he would see his girlfriend as he thought she needed counseling. Because Mr. Powers wanted the counselor to meet the girl and the counselor was not sure that she needed treatment, he agreed to see her in consultation on the question of referral. It was important for the counselor to respond to Mr. Powers' request as he was finding it difficult to trust people but did have confidence in his counselor. The counselor saw Mr. Powers' girlfriend for consultation about referral because he felt that a simple referral would be interpreted by Mr. Powers as lack of concern.

> Mr. Finch, age 38, was very suspicious that his wife was having an affair with his best friend. Ms. Finch had asked the counselor for an appointment as she was having headaches and insomnia. The counselor

refused to see her because he thought it might add to Mr. Finch's paranoia. The counselor did make a referral that was acceptable to the couple.

PHOTOGRAPHS AND ART WORK

Some clients will bring photographs of themselves or their family for the counselor to see. It is easy to look at the photographs and return them. If the client wants the counselor to keep the pictures, the counselor returns them, explaining that it is preferable for the client to keep them since they belong to him. Ordinarily, the counselor need not make any comments about the photographs other than to remark that they are very interesting. If there has been a dramatic change in the client's appearance, the counselor may want to ask about it.

When a client brings in his own art work, he expects some comment from the counselor. The counselor explores the client's motivation for showing the art work with a question such as "What prompted you to bring this in?" If the counselor genuinely feels that the work is worthy of praise, a compliment is appropriate. Also, the client may have wished to show that he was capable of completing a task. However, the focus belongs on the client's understanding what prompted him to bring his work to the session.

Working on understanding such actions can be useful, especially if they are repeated. Through exploration the client may learn that he is bringing photos and art work to the sessions as a distraction or form of resistance. At times, at the end of the counseling, a client may want to give the counselor a piece of his work as a remembrance. If there is no reason to believe that the relationship will resume at a later date, such a gift is appropriate and can be accepted.

REFERENCES

1. Schubert M: Interviewing in Social Work Practice: An Introduction. New York, Council on Social Work Education, 1971

7

TYPICAL CLINICAL SYNDROMES

There are a variety of clients whose styles of relating to the world represent basic defense mechanisms. Their methods of relating to a counselor reflect their customary ways of responding to others or dealing with their life problems. This chapter distinguishes certain clinical syndromes for diagnostic purposes. Such diagnostic understanding of the individual gives direction for treatment techniques.

THE INTELLECTUALIZING CLIENT

The intellectualizing client has generally read several books on counseling or has avidly gleaned some knowledge of counseling from movies, friends in counseling, or other sources. This client, in telling the counselor about the problem, uses language and tone that resemble formulations being presented in a formal seminar. These presentations are without any affect and seem as though they might be about someone else. Despite this, if one listens carefully, such formulations sometimes contain a great deal of useful information about the client.

In time, when the counselor and client get to know each other, this manner of dealing with conflict may partially relax. If an interchange with the counselor or some other key figure is experienced as traumatic, the intellectualizing reappears and may be the first signal the counselor gets of the client's renewed anxiety. If such a client, with no warning, suddenly permits the outbreak of strong feelings or direct anxiety, it usually is a sign of difficulty.

Mr. Allen, a 27-year old taxi driver who had had two years of graduate work in history, came in with the chief complaint of many years of difficulty in relating to people. This difficulty became acute when a woman whom he regarded as a potential girlfriend told him that he was too cold. Although his feelings were hurt, he knew that he presented himself as very distant. Mr. Allen decided to investigate what made him that way and called the clinic for an appointment. Typically, he then went to the library to get several books on the subject of people who could not feel.

After telling the counselor of his "research," Mr. Allen proceeded to take two sheets of paper with long quotes on them from his pocket and began to read them to the counselor. The counselor said that he thought perhaps they could learn more if the client told him what he felt about himself in his own words. The client looked blank, put the papers away, and then launched into a description of the dynamics of the compulsive personality, drawn from Fenichel and Noyes. The counselor asked the client if his desire to describe himself in so scholarly a fashion was natural for him or was because he did not quite know how to handle the therapeutic situation. The client was surprised by this question and after a second or two admitted that he did often answer people with a good deal of technical detail. In fact, he indicated that he had dropped out of graduate school because several instructors had told him that he could repeat work from books accurately enough but added few of his own ideas.

The counselor successfully conveyed to the client that his desire to intellectualize, i.e., repeat material obtained from books without permitting these thoughts contact with his own ideas and feelings, was consistent throughout his life. This was the beginning of an effort to enable the client to see the intellectualizing itself as a problem so that client and counselor could both notice it and point it out without the client feeling threatened and becoming resentful.

A 25-year-old woman who was a poet came to find out why she was unable to feel close to her husband. She told the counselor that she and her husband had recently moved to a commune, and she extolled the communal life. The counselor asked her if the move to communal living was a way of avoiding closeness to her husband. The client denied that any problems with her husband had influenced her in the decision to go live with a group. Instead, she repeated the advantages and virtues of communal life. She went on to talk about her dissatisfaction with mores of today's society. She described the number of people she knew who were trapped in unsatisfactory jobs and loveless marriages just like her parents, who were afraid to make any changes or moves. The counselor asked the client if she knew that not everyone in this society agreed with her. The client was annoyed by this question and restated that the only hope for people was through communal living. She still wanted to argue about the evils of current social conventions and left the interview looking unhappy.

Here the counselor, rather than bypassing the intellectualized content in the discussions of society and concentrating on the client's discomfort about her difficulty in feeling close to anyone, incorrectly chose to enter into discussions of these intellectual constructs. As a result, the client was forced to defend her ideas, which she could only do by falling back on her customary defense, even though the defense was, in a sense, a symptom of her problem.

THE INGRATIATING CLIENT

The ingratiating client attempts to please the counselor by saying, doing, or even at times thinking what he imagines is expected of him. Such clients frequently agree too readily with what the counselor says, search out examples of behavior or thought that will show how much they have been helped by the counseling, or report incidents where others have told them how the counseling has bettered them.

The client's zeal to please the counselor prevents him from being interested in himself and interferes with his taking a realistic look at what is going on in his inner and outer life. By simply pleasing the counselor or imitating him, the client hopes to absorb a ready-made solution to his difficulties and thus avoid the therapeutic process. The counselor recognizes the anxiety that goes into this desire to please. He tries to make the client recognize that these reports of improvement and agreement with whatever the counselor says actually indicate the principal problem and do not result in much actual change in the client's life. If this clarification is rejected, the counselor can usually show the client how little desire he has to end the relationship or to accept the improvements as a conclusion of the job at hand.

Mr. Cox came to therapy because of marital problems. He told the counselor that he and his wife loved each other and their four children very much. However, his wife felt he tried too hard to be a "good boy" and was too passive. Because that seemed unmanly to her she had lost all sexual interest in him. He was unable to understand this and told the counselor how proud he was of the fact that he had many friends and had always done well at his job. The counselor showed Mr. Cox how often he talked about the good things he did and wondered how much importance he placed on being good. Mr. Cox thanked the counselor for showing him these things because he was sure that that was what bothered his wife.

The next week he came in and repeated how helpful he found the counselor's comment and then went on to describe how friendly he had gotten with some students who attended a demonstration he had given. His description of how much the students liked him was similar to many descriptions he had given in the past. The counselor asked Mr. Cox if his expression of appreciation the previous week might have been more a wish to please the counselor than an expression of interest in the issue of wanting to be good. Mr. Cox was a bit taken aback by this question and defended his sincerity. The counselor then pointed out that the client's current story showed no awareness that his trying so hard to please was a problem. For the first time in their relationship Mr. Cox became annoyed and said that he was only reporting what had actually happened.

No counselor desires to annoy his clients. However, in Mr. Cox's case his annoyance arose not because the counselor did something provocative or unpleasant. It occurred because the client's standard effort to be ingratiating, which worked well for him in casual relationships but poorly in close ones, was threatened by the therapeutic clarification. By permitting himself annoyance, Mr. Cox began to see the counselor as a threat to his loved-hated style of creating interpersonal relationships rather than as just one more person to be beguiled. The counselor knew that it would take a long time for Mr. Cox to recognize that being pleasing or friendly at *all* times to virtually *all* people was not the warm human gesture that he hoped it to be. This could only be made clear to Mr. Cox within the actual interview situation where he might slowly be able to see that his superficial appreciation of the counselor distanced them from each other. It was in an odd way defeating to the therapeutic process and thus, in Mr. Cox's eyes, to the counselor.

THE SEDUCTIVE CLIENT

The seductive client wants to win the counselor for his or her own. Some proprietary interest in the therapist, which probably occurs in every treatment, should not be confused with the interest expressed by the truly seductive client. The therapeutic situation is threatened when the client sees his or her sexual interest in the counselor as a rational desire. Such a view is apt to occur when the counselor is seen as more attractive or able to offer more satisfaction than other figures in the client's life. The wish for gratification from the counselor can be detrimental to the client as the hope and effort for a demonstration override his interest in self-examination and self-understanding. The counselor constantly shows the client how these wishes need to be discussed and understood, not gratified.

There are clients who would feel satisfied only if they could achieve an overt sexual relationship with the counselor. However, it is more usual for the client to try to overcome some less stringent boundary of the therapeutic situation. In either case, the client's energy goes into efforts at whatever represents seduction. Unless the counselor recognizes the situation early and clarifies the wasted effort and the transference involved for the client, the counselor's efforts are sidetracked into resisting cajolery. This may be anxiety-provoking for the beginning counselor, who is diverted from the task at hand.

Mr. and Ms. Storey, whose son had been hospitalized for schizophrenia, began to see a young female counselor. After only two meetings Mr. Storey suggested that the counselor get her husband and that they all go out to dinner. The counselor responded by saying that she did not consider that a productive way to work. The issue subsided for a time until the counselor decided to see Mr. and Ms. Storey separately.

Alone with the counselor, Mr. Storey began to tell her of his series of extramarital affairs. Over several interviews he recounted his disappointment with each partner, ending up with the announcement that he really cared for the counselor and felt that she alone could offer him the satisfaction he sought. She told him that this would not happen and that they would talk about it more. However, instead of putting the situation into a more direct therapeutic context by showing Mr. Storey ways to explore his own responses to her and other women, the counselor found herself defensively telling him that she as a counselor would not participate as he wished.

In this case, Mr. Storey's advances caused the counselor considerable anxiety. By reacting defensively her comments were not seen as neutral by the client. He saw her response as a challenge. Although the client might consider any type of refusal a challenge, the challenge would be minimized if the counselor showed the client in a straightforward way that he often had such wishes. He and the counselor could then explore these wishes in proper perspective and in a way that would benefit the client.

> In her third interview, Ms. Fisher, who was 28 years old, attractive, and unmarried, began to tell the counselor of her sexual experiences and exploits in some detail. After a while the counselor asked what she was trying to understand from these stories. She said that the counselor knew that she had never had a satisfactory experience with a man and that she wanted some explanation. When the counselor was quiet through the rest of this recital, she became downcast. At the beginning of the next session, Ms. Fisher told the counselor that he had seemed cold and unfeeling about her troubles with men and this had depressed her. She asked him to please talk to her more and to offer some advice as to how to deal with one of the men she currently knew. It was very upsetting to her to be away from this boyfriend, yet their relationship was very unsatisfactory when they were together. The counselor wondered about the request for advice and asked her what expectations she had from such advice. Ms. Fisher became angry and again called the counselor cold and distant. He observed that she was apparently often disappointed in him. She agreed vehemently. He asked her if she understood her disappointment in him—if it was because he was unable to work with her about her upsetting emotional conflicts, if it was due to his not giving her advice, or if it was a more general problem of his not operating in a way similar to what she had experienced with many earlier figures in her life. She broke into tears and admitted that she had wanted to sit in his lap from the first time they met and had, until this moment, believed that this expression of closeness would allow her to truly feel better.

THE CIRCUMSTANTIAL CLIENT

Some clients find it very difficult to describe anything specifically. They go around and around, describing events in half-finished phrases and sweeping generalizations, making it difficult for the counselor to understand what they are trying to say. If the counselor asks too forcefully for details, these clients either become even more abstract and wordy or respond with details so minuscule that again no salient information emerges.

> Ms. Sanders, age 24, sought treatment because of a depression following an abortion. She said she was alone much of the time and felt cut off from people. The counselor asked her what her parents were like and later asked about her previous relationships with boyfriends and girlfriends. Ms. Sanders responded by telling him in great detail that her parents were wonderful people. She went on to say repetitiously how good they were and how sorry she was to be so much trouble to them. The counselor again asked what sort of person her father was and got a response identical to the first one. At the end of the hour the counselor felt he had learned little about the client. He knew only that she had had the abortion and that it was a terrible experience, but he did not know what had made it so hard for her.
>
> When the same sort of interaction continued during the second hour, the counselor asked if Ms. Sanders was frightened at seeing him. At first she denied it but then admitted that she was afraid of being criticized and feeling exposed. The counselor asked how she responded to such situations. She had no idea. He pursued it, asking her if perhaps when anxious she threw out a smoke screen of words; he asked her if this had happened to her at other times. At first Ms. Sanders was puzzled, but then she told him how the boys in the apartment next door to her teased her about never finishing a thought.

In this case the counselor resisted pressing for details, asking for definitions of vague words, or attempting to discuss abstract ideas when he understood little of what Ms. Sanders was talking about. Instead, he tried to interest her in her own condition. As long as he could get part of her to observe her fear of exposure with him, they could communicate with each other.

THE QUESTIONING CLIENT

Some clients, at the beginning or during the course of a therapeutic relationship, find it important to question the counselor closely. Sometimes these questions are obviously inappropriate, but more often clients select areas to question where they feel their questions justified. The justification may come from the intensity of their wish for answers from the counselor or may come because they feel the content of the question appropriate to the counselor's area of expertise. Hence, they feel the question reasonable and expect an answer.

Such questions as "How are we doing?" "Do you think we have accomplished anything today?" "What would you do in a spot like this?" "What should I do about my friend who is having trouble?" and "I'm stuck, where do we go from here?" are extremely common. The extensive publicity, particularly cartoons and jokes, about counselors make it difficult for the counselor to simply throw the question back. The technique of merely reflecting back the client's comments has always had its limitations even if only used sparingly. Nevertheless, the client knows that many apparently sensible and realistic questions, as well as all the others, conceal latent wishes. They are asked for reasons very different from those that can be seen in the manifest inquiry and cannot simply be met with silence.

> Mr. Wald, a 20-year-old college student, sought out a counselor because of compulsive handwashing, fear of sexual deviance, and inability to live comfortably outside the family home. A few minutes after meeting the counselor, he began to ask questions, among them, "Should I force myself to live away from home?" and "Should I tell my father about the counseling?" The counselor met the onslaught by pointing out that Mr. Wald seemed to want many rules and regulations. The client agreed enthusiastically with this comment, stating that he himself was full of doubts and expected direction from the counseling. When the counselor asked Mr. Wald what made it difficult for him to select a direction for himself, he said that was the counselor's job to determine. He went on to say that the counselor had not answered his questions. The counselor asked if Mr. Wald would first elaborate his views about counseling and how it worked. Mr. Wald was able to give a coherent account of what counseling was: he was supposed to talk freely and try to understand his motives. The counselor agreed, adding information about the shared nature of the work and pointing out that understanding the reasons for asking the questions was often a very important part of counseling. Mr. Wald went along with this and then elaborated for a few minutes about his home situation. Suddenly he stopped and said again that the counselor had to tell him what to say to his father. "You don't know what a critical guy he is," Mr. Wald said. "You must tell me what to say to him or he won't let me come back." The counselor told Mr. Wald that he was most sympathetic to his situation but did not know what the father should be told. Mr. Wald accepted this announcement of ignorance with reluctance and left.

The next time he began the hour by asking the counselor how long the counseling would take, adding that the counselor should certainly know the answer to that. The counselor said that he now knew Mr. Wald well enough to know that understanding what went into his asking questions was more important than any answer could be. Mr. Wald was clearly unhappy with this answer but continued the counseling, beginning and ending every interview with a question.

Until client and counselor together could understand more thoroughly what Mr. Wald wanted unconsciously from the counselor, Mr. Wald would probably have to continue to ask questions. The counselor tried to find a way to interest Mr. Wald in his question asking and yet not answer his question. Although it was frustrating to Mr. Wald not to have his questions answered, little therapeutic work would be accomplished if the counselor offered answers to the manifest content and ignored the underlying wishes. By giving the client answers to all of his questions, the counselor would be pretending to an expertise that neither he nor anyone else had. The difficult part was to refuse to answer Mr. Wald's questions without criticizing him for asking them. As long as Mr. Wald could feel the counselor working with him, albeit on the questioning rather than on the questions, he found the frustration tolerable.

THE ENTITLED CLIENT

Some people grow up with a conviction that life must be fair (mainly to them); it is a way of thinking that is normal for the young child, who feels he has certain "rights" and is outraged when they are violated. These clients imagine they must inhibit and restrict their wishes and desires until as adults they still believe that they are absolutely entitled to certain satisfactions. Once convinced that a particular desire fits into their scheme of fairness, they not only expect the desire to be fulfilled, but feel it is important to do anything in their power to obtain it and can easily find reasons for their behavior that make a guilty conscience unnecessary. The particular desire then has both intellectual and emotional backing from within the client, who thus experiences very little, if any, conflict. This "backing" may leave little room for the counselor, who wants to give the client a chance to question this sense of entitlement without feeling criticized or becoming defensive.

> Mr. Washington, age 30, had sought counseling because of a growing awareness that he was afraid of his wife. After two months of treatment, he brought his wife to an appointment. He asked the counselor to see them together and to convince his wife to go to a counselor herself. The counselor insisted on talking to Mr. Washington alone, with the aim of showing him that he could not make such a recommendation without knowing his wife. He also felt it was important to understand how Mr. Washington had decided on this course of action. The client would have none of it. He told his counselor that months had gone by and that his fear of his wife was unabated. In a self-righteous rage he pointed out that he had come to the sessions on time, paid his bills, and now wanted a return on his investment. It became clear that Mr. Washington would accept no rational argument that asked him to look at his behavior. The counselor asked him when he first thought of bringing his wife with him. Mr. Washington was a bit taken aback and said that he had thought of it that very morning. The counselor pointed out that in their first interview the client had asked him if he "wanted" to see his wife. Although Mr. Washington denied this, the counselor could see that some of the fire had gone out of him about this episode. The counselor asked Mr. Washington if he had not always expected that the counselor would step in and handle this frightening woman and if this was not part of the pattern of passivity that had brought him into treatment in the first place. Mr. Washington answered that he felt disappointed and let down. The counselor sympathized with his disappointment but then said that his wishes that the counselor bail him out were very much a part of the treatment. The problem had become acute because he was now demanding that his wishes be fulfilled, rather than examining the basis for his wishes.

In order to explore the situation, the counselor focused on Mr. Washington's interest in building a case to justify himself since this was more important than the client's original wishes about his wife. The counselor specifically asked Mr. Washington to notice what incidents triggered off the underlying conviction of entitlement so that they could get to the root of it. Otherwise, the client would repeatedly find himself in an uncomfortable position either because his demands inevitably led to frustration or because he did not discover his demands and became angry with himself for his passivity.

THE INSATIABLE CLIENT

There are clients who are never satisfied, and these same people tolerate delay poorly. Frequently these are the clients who repeatedly telephone the counselor, who have trouble leaving the appointment, and who expect immediate attention when troubled. They are often terribly sensitive to what they see as rejection, and their feelings are easily hurt. Here the counselor must find a way to make explicit to the client that his need for immediate gratification is excessive. Because the client will require some gratification, the counselor must also find a way to preserve reasonable therapeutic boundaries without causing the client undue pain. The boundaries are necessary because the counselor knows that these clients' demands are infinite. The counselor also knows that these clients become more anxious and guilt-ridden if they fear that these powerful impulses are uncontrollable. The demands and fears are confirmed if the counselor does not set clear limits. The counselor's ability to maintain limits and to protect himself indicate to the client that his insatiable demands can be resisted and managed.

Ms. Sawyer, a 24-year-old graduate student, sought treatment because of increasing difficulty in studying and a long series of unsatisfactory relationships with men. During her first two interviews she spoke easily, chiefly supplying history. Although Ms. Sawyer constantly looked to the counselor for cues, she could proceed without them. A few days after the second interview, she met a man who again seemed to be "it." At that point Ms. Sawyer became extremely anxious and began to call the counselor four to ten times each night asking for advice on how to handle the relationship and reassurance that she was not going to be rejected again. Her therapeutic hours became the same as the phone calls, most of the time being spent with Ms. Sawyer begging for help. The counselor tried to show her that she experienced her wish for this man as a need as intense as the feeling of a man dying of thirst on the desert. He repeated this clarification and made other appropriate analogies.

The counselor's efforts were devoted to showing the client the difference between a real need or danger and the exaggerated feeling of need or danger experienced by someone who wants something badly and may not get it. Slowly Ms. Sawyer began to understand that her sense of urgency was irrational and excessive and that human relationships were interactive and not the same as food for the starving. For a time this awareness reduced her feelings of helplessness that led to her total demands. After a while her relationship again became everything to her, and once more she felt that the counselor had to help her preserve it immediately and at all times. Each new wave of urgency eventually yielded to the counselor's clarifications and each remission lasted a bit longer, but it was a difficult struggle.

THE INHIBITED CLIENT

Some clients present a lifelong history of shyness and lack of confidence. They worry that they will be easily embarrassed or will give the "wrong" impression if they behave at all forthrightly. They are fearful that they will be misunderstood and that their feelings will be hurt. Of equal concern to them is their fear that they may hurt or offend others. Their history usually reveals how this lack of confidence interfered with their functioning in usual childhood activities, such as speaking in class or participating in a school play or various games, and then continued into adolescence as an obstacle to group activities and dating. In many cases, counseling had been contemplated before, but the symptom itself prevented them from taking that step. For people with so much overt concern about revealing themselves, the idea of talking freely to another human being is, in itself, frightening. Hence, the initial therapeutic problem is not so much to uncover deep-seated conflicts but to work with the discomfort so that the client can tolerate counseling.

Whether this shyness is a generalized concern with the world and its inhabitants or a way of expressing a more specific phobia often cannot be decided until the client knows what specifically stimulates the inhibition. With sexual inhibitions, in particular, it may turn out that the overall characterological response may be only a part of the issue and a more specific fear about sexuality may be the more intrinsic problem.

At her first interview Ms. Barnard, age 23, spoke haltingly and with much embarrassment about her trouble in expressing herself since early childhood. In response to a question, she indicated that her behavior in the interview was typical. When the counselor asked about her social and sexual history, she blushed and was unable to answer. After a brief silence, the counselor went on to ask about her father's occupation. Ms. Barnard remained tongue-tied and then began to cry. She told the counselor with great difficulty that she was sorry she had come, that she knew she could not do it, and that she hated to be so stupid. He asked her what made her feel that way. Ms. Barnard said that she knew she would not be able to answer his questions and would fail at this as she had at other attempts at relationships. The counselor sympathized with her discomfort but pointed out that she was not being realistic. She had after all answered all of his questions until that point, and therefore they had learned something about what set her off. Also, since she had been shy much of her life, she must have anticipated that the same issues would come up in counseling. In fact, she could only hope to work with these problems if they showed themselves. Ms. Barnard was impressed with the logic of the counselor's remarks but told him that she was not sure that she could stand the discomfort. He pointed out that her discussion of her discomfort was quite straightforward and that it ought to permit her a bit more self-confidence. She left the office considerably more cheerful than when she had arrived.

Mr. Calder, age 27, sought treatment because he felt unable to form relationships with women and, in fact, could hardly call a woman for a date. When he did call, he had an agonizing time. He was shy during the therapeutic sessions but managed to talk about his problems with only minor discomfort except when the discussion turned to sex. Then Mr. Calder turned beet red and began to stammer. The counselor suggested that he had very specific concerns in the area of sex that were different from his general fears of making a fool of himself. Mr. Calder nodded but was unable to speak. The counselor asked him if he felt that his thoughts were sufficiently unusual or difficult that even a counselor would think him terribly strange. Again Mr. Calder could only nod. The counselor said that it was important for him to realize that counselors are not there to judge but to make sense of things. Although he did not know the details of his fantasies, the counselor would wager that they were not as unusual as the client apparently imagined. After this Mr. Calder brightened and told of the extent of his anxiety when in the presence of an eligible woman. Thus, the client began to open up about his conflicts to make them accessible to examination and future resolution.

DRUG PROBLEMS

Clients with serious drug problems, usually involving opiates, barbiturates, or amphetamines, only rarely come to the attention of a counselor on their own. Usually they end up in a clinic or a hospital as a result of the insistence of others, are brought in by the police, or are brought in as a result of passing out or having an accident while drugged. This is in sharp contrast to the drug experimenter who after an anxiety-arousing experience with marijuana or a psychedelic drug often wants to talk over his reaction with a professional.

Like some alcoholics, the heavy drug user finds it hard to face the reality of his life and tends to tell the interviewer a life story that seems more palatable at the moment. In contrast to the alcoholic, the drug user is more likely to magnify his use of drugs. Those who are drug-dependent find it almost impossible to maintain a therapeutic relationship unless they are in a drug-maintenance situation as outpatients or, if they are willing to try abstinence, in a living-in situation specially designed for them.

However, there are two groups of drug users worth emphasizing. The first is the group who have become drug-dependent because of a wish to be responsible rather than irresponsible. Their initial drug use began because of a medical problem—to eliminate pain, get sleep, or get energy in order to be able to function. They often cannot bear their drug dependency, and their hope to overcome it permits them to form an alliance with a counselor.

The second is a group of people who have tried and used almost all drugs and present themselves as multiple drug users. But on close examination their drug use is seen to be only a way of presenting themselves or defending themselves against personal difficulties and should not be permitted to act as a smoke screen to draw the focus away from their troubles.

> Ms. Norfolk, age 34, was referred by an internist for counseling because she was demanding more and more amphetamines. Two years earlier she had been given low doses to help with a diet. When her initial prescription ran out, Ms. Norfolk had not lost any weight and stopped taking the pills. One month later she felt unusually blue and asked her doctor for more of the amphetamines because they had helped when she felt logy and out of sorts. Ms. Norfolk had been on the pills ever since.
>
> The counselor observed that Ms. Norfolk was a restless woman who made many nervous movements. After just a few minutes of discussion she began to cry and told the counselor that she had bribed her druggist to give her more pills and was taking heavy doses of amphetamines daily. She said that she had to have them or she could not get through the day. "I have a husband and four children to take care of," she

almost screamed, "and I can't do it without the pills." Ms. Norfolk told a life story of wanting to be responsible, active, and worthwhile while always being convinced that she was none of these things. The counselor pointed out that she had wanted so much to be good and to do the right thing all her life and now this desire had gotten her off the track.

After two interviews she and the counselor agreed that it would take a long time to understand how she had gotten in such a fix, and they decided to meet regularly for an indefinite period.

Mr. Storrow, age 19, was admitted to the psychiatric ward of a general hospital because he had passed out following an argument with a friend. During the argument he had become agitated and had taken barbiturates. He could not remember anything after that. A friend brought him to the hospital.

Although a little groggy, Mr. Storrow felt well enough to talk the following morning. He reported using a number of drugs, including heroin, from the time he was 14. When asked what had happened when he was 14, Mr. Storrow said it was bad then because his mother had died and his father had remarried. After trying unsuccessfully to break up the marriage, he left home. He went to his sister's, but after a fight there, he ran away. Forced into a foster home, he again ran away. The last two years had been the best in his life because he had his own apartment and could get away from people. The counselor indicated that she understood how much he wanted to get away from fights and unpleasantness and wondered if that was not behind his pill taking. . After an initial denial Mr. Storrow said that that made some sense. He then told the counselor that he was very anxious to leave his job as an aide in a hospital because there were so many arguments among the members of the staff.

Mr. Storrow said that he was taking barbiturates regularly but not using any other drugs. He added that many of his friends used more drugs than he did. Also, he said that he was glad to have had the fight the night before because that friend had wanted to move in with him and he now knew it would not work. The counselor said that it was good to know that in advance. She then asked Mr. Storrow if he was concerned that he had to get away from trouble so badly that he had not even known how many pills he had taken. Mr. Storrow admitted concern but said he did not know what to do. The counselor suggested that they meet regularly to discuss it but added that she was afraid that at the first sign of difficulty he would run off. He agreed that this was likely to happen but said that he would like to try talking about it with her, and they made another appointment.

THE OVERTLY HOSTILE CLIENT

Clients express direct anger at counselors (1) because of the external circumstances that led to the therapeutic meeting; (2) because of the client's reaction to the counselor; and (3) because these feelings of anger have been displaced from another source onto the counselor. In each instance, it is most important that the counselor not respond angrily or defensively to the client's hostility. Then, at the proper time, the counselor attempts to see if he and the client can discover and make some sense out of what made the client so angry. The counselor might have been at fault and, if so, he must face this with the client.

The chief problem with the overtly hostile client is timing. The counselor does not wish to "explain away" the anger before he and the client are certain that the client's position has had a full hearing. The too-ready explanation may only add fuel to the fire or leave the client feeling simply turned off. However, if the counselor does not at some point respond to the anger, the client may become too anxious or feel that the counselor's refusal to respond is a form of retaliation.

> At his wife's insistence, Mr. Park, age 45, called the clinic for an appointment with a counselor. During the initial telephone conversation he said that his wife thought he could not get along with people, including his own children, because he was only interested in himself. She threatened to leave him unless he went to a counselor.
>
> As soon as he entered the office Mr. Park told the counselor that he was only there to get his wife off his back. Then he asked how much the clinic was charging him for this visit. When he was told the amount, he became extremely angry and asked the counselor in an aggressive tone if he thought it was worth that much money just for somebody to listen to him for an hour. The counselor asked him if he had been in treatment before and if he had any ideas about how counseling worked. This remark infuriated the client further. He told the counselor that he thought the whole thing was a racket and that his wife had been seeing a counselor for a year and that was what had started the trouble. "She's analyzing everything, including me," he shouted, "and that is as much of that shit as I plan to take from her or you." The counselor simply listened as Mr. Park went on to say how much the counseling cost, including babysitters, and how it had done more harm than good. This went on for about 10 minutes before the counselor felt it was the right time to tell Mr. Park that he did not think Mr. Park knew him well enough to be this angry with him personally. Mr. Park was still angry

enough to say that all counselors are part of the same slimy pack. The counselor said that he realized the client was unhappy with his wife's treatment and that they could talk about his complaints and added that counselors were not there just to defend each other. "Maybe not, but you'll probably just ask me questions about me and not help me with my wife's preoccupation with her shrink," Mr. Park replied. The counselor was forced to smile and agree with Mr. Park, but he went on to say that if Mr. Park could better understand himself, he would know more about his reactions to his wife and the counselor in this difficult situation. The counselor pointed out that they could discuss his opinions and feelings about his wife's counseling, but they could not discuss the counseling itself since that would be pure guesswork. However, he again assured Mr. Park that he had no wish to defend the other counselor. Mr. Park was somewhat mollified and told the counselor to go on with his questions. The counselor said he would but quickly added that there was not much time left and asked how angry Mr. Park would be about coming back again.

In this case Mr. Park had been coerced into seeing a counselor. Furthermore, he was already furious with his wife's counselor, and this anger he easily displaced onto his counselor, who correctly saw no need to defend his colleague. Since it had become apparent to the counselor that Mr. Park had a low boiling point, the counselor not only wanted to help Mr. Park make sense of his response during the interview, but by his last comment to prepare Mr. Park for future events that might also make him angry. By taking up the possibility of anger in advance, the counselor hoped to give the client a vantage point from which to question more closely what made him so angry.

Ms. Morris, whose 18-year-old son had recently been admitted to a psychiatric hospital, was referred by the hospital for an appointment with a counselor. She was asked numerous questions about her family and her son's early development. When Ms. Morris wanted to know how this information was going to be used, the counselor asked her why she wanted to know. Ms. Morris replied that she had been told almost nothing about what they were going to do for her son. She felt someone should tell her something. The counselor asked Ms. Morris how she felt about her son being in the hospital. "Terrible," she replied "and worse every minute because pipsqueaks like you sit there and ask stupid questions and never tell me anything." You sound angry because your son is here," said the counselor. "No, I feel sick because he is here, but angry at you for picking on me and not answering my questions. I don't even know what medicine he's taking. What is it?" "Are you afraid that we will give him something that is not good for him?" asked the counselor. At that Ms. Morris began to cry with rage and just screamed at the counselor that he was an inhuman monster who had no idea what it meant to be on the other side of the desk and see a loved one be admitted to a psychiatric hospital. Ms. Morris went on for some time, and the counselor was visibly shaken. When Ms. Morris's crying had subsided, the counselor apologized and said that indeed he could and should answer some of her questions, but that it was important to know how she felt about such an event. He had just done the wrong thing first, he admitted. The mother calmed down and asked and received answers to some of her questions. However, before she left the hospital she asked the administration if she could see a different counselor the next time she came.

Mr. Redfield, a 22-year-old college senior, had been seeing a counselor for three months. On one occasion he arrived for his regular weekly appointment in a rage. A paper on which he had worked for weeks had been returned to him that day, and he felt that he had been unfairly treated and that Professor Alter had long been down on him and "was a bastard." Mr. Redfield had been venting his spleen about Professor Alter for some time when the counselor asked him what his grade had been.

Mr. Redfield: The grade doesn't matter as much as the professor not paying any attention to my work. Like all smart bastards of professors, he just does what he has to do and doesn't give a damn about the students.

Counselor: What did you get?

Mr. Redfield: B.

Counselor: Is that so bad?

Mr. Redfield: Yes, considering the work I put in.

There was a strained silence, finally broken by the counselor who asked if Mr. Redfield had talked the matter over with Professor Alter.

Mr. Redfield: I wouldn't give that bastard another chance.

Counselor: Another chance? Have you talked to him before?

Mr. Redfield: Yes, he was my instructor in a course in my second year.

Counselor: How did that go?

Mr. Redfield: Well, I started off with an A, and I used to go in and talk to him a lot. That was before I knew he wasn't interested. Then I turned in a long paper and got a C, and when I talked it over with him, he told me I was lucky to get a C as it was, but he had given me a C because he thought that it was his fault for helping me too much and not letting me develop my own ideas. He would have let me rewrite the paper, but who wanted to do that?

Counselor: What had you expected?

Mr. Redfield: Well, I thought we were good friends and that if he didn't like the paper he would talk to me about it and not stick a knife in me. That's when I got mad.

Counselor: And yet you're taking another course with him. You must have felt something other than rage.

Mr. Redfield: Not when I found out what a bastard he was.

Counselor: How about before?

Mr. Redfield: Well, for a while I thought he was the first friend I had made on the faculty. I should have known better.

Counselor: You sound more sad than mad now.

Mr. Redfield: Well, you know how out of it I was my first year. Then in my second year I began to put it together a little and meeting Professor Alter made me feel great. I thought we would really be friends. When he treated me this way, it really knocked the pins out from under me.

Counselor: You took the course this year because you still had hopes?

Mr. Redfield: I guess so. How silly can you get?

Counselor: Not silly, just not letting yourself know how much you wanted from this man and thus assuring yourself a disappointment and an excuse to get mad all over again.

THE ALCOHOLIC CLIENT

In general, the client with a serious drinking problem either does not make his own appointment with a counselor or quickly indicates that someone else had insisted that he do so. It is not that he is entirely unaware that he has a serious problem. Rather, he is so sure that he can do nothing about it that he wants above all to avoid the shame that arises from being exposed as helpless. Hence, he cannot acknowledge to anyone except his secret self the seriousness of the situation.

The different patterns of problem drinking are not described here, but whether the client is a daily drinker, a spree drinker, or another kind, he tends to minimize his drinking to the counselor. He may apologetically admit that his wife thinks he drinks too much but will go on to insist that he has control over the situation.

Many authorities regard alcoholism as a defense against an underlying chronic depression. Sometimes, after an interview or two, the heavy-drinking client indicates that besides the depression that may have preceded the drinking, but that certainly accompanies it, he suffers from acute anxiety about a specific personal conflict. In some situations he may be able to continue in a therapeutic situation. More often it becomes clear to the counselor that until the client has stopped drinking, no real therapeutic interaction is possible. In those cases the counselor is likely to arrange a mutually agreed upon referral to Alcoholics Anonymous or to another association or institution instead of continuing a counseling relationship.

> When Ms. Tobin telephoned the clinic for an appointment for her husband, she was asked if her husband could call for himself. Ms. Tobin said that her husband did not believe that his drinking necessitated his going to a clinic. She could not understand how he could be so blind since he had lost his job, been brought home by police numerous times, lost his driver's license, and hurt his back twice from falling, all while drunk. Because Ms. Tobin had valid reasons for calling, she was given an appointment for her husband for the next week. If Mr. Tobin agreed to come in, Ms. Tobin was requested to tell him to please not drink on the day of the appointment.
>
> Mr. Tobin arrived on time for the appointment, but as soon as he entered the office the smell of liquor on his breath was apparent. However, he spoke coherently throughout and was obviously an intelligent, sophisticated person. In response to questions he admitted some daily alcohol consumption but insisted that his wife exaggerated the amount. His recent difficulties were ascribed to a run of hard luck, and he spoke confidently of a change for the better. He had drunk too much on a few occasions, but that was in the past, and he had learned better. The family history revealed that his mother had been a heavy drinker and had been hospitalized for detoxification on numerous occasions. During his youth the family social and financial situation had declined sharply, and his father had died of a heart attack when Mr. Tobin was 20, just a year after his mother's death of cirrhosis of the liver. At that time Mr. Tobin had little or no communication with his brother or sister although he did not quite know how that had happened. He recognized that his marriage was now in jeopardy, and again he did not quite understand how that had happened.
>
> The counselor asked Mr. Tobin if he could explain what made his wife think he had a problem when he did not see it that way. Mr. Tobin responded by going over his hard luck story again. When pressed about how he would feel if he could not pull things together as he planned, Mr. Tobin said he "didn't know."
>
> Counselor: I think you will be so disappointed in yourself and ashamed that you might have to drink more.
>
> Mr. Tobin: No, I'll be OK this time.
>
> Counselor: If it doesn't work, will you be too embarrassed to talk to

me again? There is a lot about Alcoholics Anonymous and other organizations that I don't think you understand.

Mr. Tobin: Had friends (laugh), started to say drinking buddies, who are or were A.A. Sounds too sanctimonious for me.

Counselor: Well, maybe, but will you come to see me again?

Mr. Tobin: No need.

Counselor: Would it be OK if I called you in a month?

Mr. Tobin: That's nice of you, but you needn't bother.

Counselor: But I'll want to find out how things have gone.

After three phone calls the counselor learned that things had not gone well and that Mr. Tobin was drinking more heavily than ever. Mr. Tobin finally accepted an appointment and, when he came in this time, he looked disheveled, red-eyed, and generally debilitated. During the interview Mr. Tobin accepted a referral to A.A. and arranged to meet a member at the clinic that same afternoon.

8

THE BEGINNING COUNSELOR'S
FIRST INTERVIEW

First interviews are usually regarded as intake or evaluation sessions and require an understanding of the client's problems, an orderly assessment of his mode of personality functioning, and his goals. Initial evaluation procedures with an interviewer who is not likely to be the client's regular counselor usually are completed in one or two sessions. The client should always be told in the beginning that the evaluator will not—if this is the case—be his counselor. Despite this precaution, when the evaluation lasts for three or more interviews, a relationship of some importance may be established so that a transfer to another counselor can occasion sufficient disappointment and frustration in the client to make him uncomfortable and to interfere with the counseling.

While it is not possible for a beginner to get all the background data required, it is good to keep in mind an outline of the points to be covered. If the initial interview is clearly evaluative, then basic information includes: (1) present difficulty or chief complaint; (2) previous history of difficulty; (3) general past history, including medical and psychological difficulties; (4) family history, including specific data as to age and health of parents and siblings, their occupations and general social status, personality descriptions and their interrelationships with each other and the client; (5) social history, including lifelong friend-ship and dating patterns; (6) sexual history; and (7) current family and social situation including living arrangements, education, occu-pation, financial status, vocation, marital status, children, and so on. Generally, the interview is begun with open-ended questions, such as "What brings you here?" The client thus has the opportu-nity to present his story in his own way. The same is true when bringing up other essential parts of history. Family history, for example, can be elicited by asking, "What was your early life like?" or "Tell me about your background."

It is important before the evaluative process is over to know many facts about the client. Clients who are voluble about their current difficulty may have to be interrupted and asked specific questions. It is quite reasonable to say, "I see we only have a short time left, and it would be important to talk about your family background. Could you tell me if your parents are alive, how old they are, and so on." If the client digresses, the interviewer returns the client to the history with specific questions. This technique of interrupting to ask specific questions in a formal manner, more reminiscent of a medical than a psychological history, can be particularly useful when asking questions the interviewer fears may be embarrassing for the client. Sometimes little mention is made of sexual activity and responses or ways of dealing with anger. Instead of pointing out the omission, the counselor may prefer to interrupt and ask a straightforward question. He may begin his questions by saying, "I hope these questions are not too embarrassing, but before we get through the evaluation it is important that you talk about your sexual activities and interest." (See the section on inquiry into embarrassing subjects, in Chap. 3.) Usually clients will answer specific questions. If they indicate that the questions stir up issues too painful to discuss, the counselor rarely persists, although if the area now under discussion was not part of the original complaint, he may point out that this degree of anxiety may in itself be an important issue for the counseling.

Clients will frequently ask, "Where should I begin?" Because this often is an indication of dependency, a response such as "Wherever you like" or "It's up to you" will minimize the dependency from the outset. No matter how hard the patient searches for an accurate accounting of his past and present, it is an impossible task. Obviously, most memories are "screened" or colored by his own wishes, fantasies, daydreams, and so forth, and the reality of past events is often far different. For example, if three people are asked to give their versions of a recent argument, they will all be somewhat different depending on their vantage point as well as their biases.

In this chapter we present two first-person case reports prepared by beginning counselors after their initial interview with the client. In our discussions of these interviews every effort is made to show how they could be improved. As mentioned later, in our discussion on supervision in an actual supervising situation, few, if any, supervisors would pick up so many so-called mistakes. The supervisor would, as will the reader, be impressed by the honesty of the reports and the concern and interest implicit in them. The supervisor would convey appreciation of the work and would take up the points that seem most pertinent to the case at the moment. In future sessions the supervisor would have the chance to talk over whatever points were omitted initially, although often, with experience and help from clients, the trainee picks up many things on his own.

The first interview for the counselor may or may not be the first interview for the client. In some cases the client has already been interviewed at that agency by someone else before this interview, which is the first with this trainee. This situation is often particularly difficult for the beginner, who feels himself being compared to the previous, more experienced interviewer.

When a client has been evaluated and referred for counseling, we strongly recommend that the assigned counselor get his own history during the first interview. The client may object, saying that he has already given a history, but once the counselor points out that reading the history is quite different from hearing it, few clients continue to object (see the section on parameters of the interview, Chap. 4). When the client gives the material directly, many nuances are conveyed that are not available from a typed record. Also, hearing it tends to fix the material more securely in a counselor's mind. It could be somewhat awkward for a counselor to ask a client he has been seeing regularly for months if he has a brother or a sister, which is more likely to happen if the counselor has read the client's history than if he has heard it directly from the client.

A word should be added about how a counselor listens to the client during this process. Throughout this book, we have downplayed specific diagnoses. We believe that the use of diagnostic categories indicates a prime emphasis on discovering what is "wrong," a search for a category into which to place these difficulties, and, particularly, a concern for symptoms. To our knowledge, no practitioners believe that they should simply assess a person's troubles and not his total functioning. A preoccupation with diagnosis, particularly for the beginner, may minimize his interest in the more difficult task of determining the continuities and structures of personality functioning that indicate the way a particular individual has found to express his version of our common humanity. The task is made difficult because the client, quite understandably, emphasizes what is wrong. He does not seek counseling to discuss issues that do not bother him. Once the interviewer begins to think in terms of holistic personality trends, he listens more for them than for specific troubles. While what causes the client pain is of essential importance to the counselor, it is only one part of the personality structure he is beginning to think through.

This structure is flexible. As the interview proceeds, new information changes his views, but no information is viewed as random. What is said and, often more important, what is omitted must have a place so that the counseling process has order and regularity. Nothing is more confusing for a counselor than the feeling that the client's material is chaotic and that the counselor's responses are piecemeal, that is, each response is only to an item of the client's commentary and not to a general trend in the client's whole structure. It is therefore most important that the counselor think in terms of the client's whole personality when listening to the specific things he has to say.

FIRST INTERVIEW—A

This selection is taken from the beginning counselor's report of her first interview. The client has already had one intake interview, and this is his second appointment at the agency.

Peter, 18 years old, had come from class and was loaded down with books and other parcels. He was good-looking, but dressed in a nondescript way and spoke in a flat, somewhat controlled voice. He chose the chair in the farthest corner and sat stiffly at first. Later he relaxed somewhat, although his tone and demeanor remained contained throughout.

After general introductions, we began by discussing the material from the intake interview. I told Peter I knew he was having difficulties at home and that he wanted to move out. He nodded, and I said that I wanted to know if that was correct.

Peter said yes, he was having trouble at home, and we began talking about systems of communications and expectations between the parents on the one hand and the children on the other. Relations between his family members were never close in terms of shared confidence, and he turned outside the family for that sort of thing. In this regard Peter envied the family relationships of his girlfriend Nancy Barber, as her parents are more open and allow her a great deal of independence. Peter reported spending a great deal of time at Nancy's house despite his parents' disapproval. He feels very discouraged because he enjoys Nancy's family life and when he tries to tell his parents about it, they do not want to listen.

I wondered if Peter had any ideas about how his parents might have felt when he was comparing them unfavorably to the Barbers. Peter looked uncomfortable with the question and asked what I meant. Stumbling, I managed to say that I thought that maybe they felt defensive about his coming home and saying how he had enjoyed Nancy's family. Peter disagreed and said that they didn't believe him and that they did not want to hear about it. He felt this was consistent with their attitude and behavior toward him. On further questioning he explained that he had gone to some effort to convince his parents that he wanted their approval of his spending time with Nancy's family, although he added that he would continue to go there "with or without their blessing."

Peter described his parents as rather old-fashioned in their expectations of their children and stern in their determination to fulfill their parental duties. They feel it is their duty to prevent the children from making the same mistakes they made.

Peter said that his father seemed more receptive than his mother to his desire for more independence. His father had suggested that Peter not discuss the matter with his mother in order to avoid further arguments because his mother would not understand anyway. Peter feels that his mother still thinks of him as her "little boy." His tone at this point seemed to me somewhere between a whimper and anger. He feels that he can only approach his mother with finalized, sensible plans. Otherwise she would shout and begin to lecture him. Peter indicated that by getting up his courage he had approached his father about his plans and feelings, but his father had shut him off, saying, "I know." I commented that the pattern of communication built up over so many years would likely take some time and effort to change but didn't it seem a worthwhile thing to try? Peter hesitated and said he thought it would be difficult, although he could try. One reason for the hesitation was that by Peter's account his father seems at first to understand, but later takes his mother's side.

Peter went on to say that he is looking into a job and living arrangements that would allow him to move away from home. When he mentioned his plans to his father, he was surprised that his father had been less volatile than expected and might even go along with his plans. Peter feared the worst if his mother finds out. He still seemed to be proceeding in a practical manner, recognizing that these matters may take some time and that he would have to manage at home in the meantime.

During the discussion of Peter's plans to move out of the home, I found myself in the uncomfortable position of Peter's mother, wanting assurances that he would not act hastily. I complicated the mistake by commenting on the similarity of positions, at which point Peter drew back in his chair and looked disappointed and almost shocked. I said I was surprised at myself since Peter had sounded quite sensible in his thoughts and plans. At this he cheered up, stating, "So you do think it's a good idea." I responded that I saw nothing wrong with his intentions and hoped he would continue to apprise his father as he went along. Peter said he would certainly try.

At this point I commented that we had talked a lot about his intentions and I was wondering how he was feeling about all that was happening in his life. Peter did not answer but asked what I meant. I responded that I had a picture of what was going on outside but I wondered how he felt inside. I added that taking a step out of the home must be scary. Peter said he realized this and was attempting to prepare himself. After a short silence, I recalled my own experience and shared the guilt I had felt about not meeting my parents' expectations. That seemed to strike a responsive chord, and Peter smiled for the first time in the interview, saying, "Yes, I know what you mean." I suggested that we might explore this area in a further session, and Peter agreed. I attempted to schedule another appointment, but Peter was unsure of his next week's class schedule. He suggested that I call him sometime next week and arrange an appointment then. I said that perhaps it would be better if he called me when he knew for sure when he would have some time free. He agreed, and we arranged for him to call at 1:45 on Tuesday.

Discussion

The counselor observed that Peter chose to sit stiffly in the farthest corner, which alerted her to his anxiety and discomfort.

In an attempt to lessen Peter's discomfort, the counselor brought up her knowledge of the previous intake interview. In general, however, although clients may think they want counselors to know about them, the idea that the counselor has information from other sources increases the client's anxiety. The counselor might simply have said that she knew an intake interview had been held, but that she preferred to work with information directly between the two of them so that she could understand just how Peter felt about things.

Next the counselor asked if her information was correct, which implied a desire to check up instead of wanting Peter to elaborate his feelings and conflicts about moving away from home. It is unclear whether the issue of expectations arose from the counselor or from the client, but since expectations are a significant area to explore, it would be important to know their source.

When the counselor asked Peter about how his parents might have felt when he compared them unfavorably to the Barbers, she came too close to judging what Peter was doing instead of trying to understand how Peter felt in the situation. Also, there was a hint of moralistic disapproval of Peter's behavior. By her next comment, the counselor confirmed her disapproval of Peter's behavior by again talking to him, not about what was going on in him, but about how his parents may have felt. If the counselor found that area to be of such importance, it would have been better to simply ask neutrally, "What happened when you discussed your relationship with the Barbers at home?" Peter went on to say that he would defy his parents if they disapproved of his relationship with the Barbers. It would not be too great a jump to imagine that he was talking about the counselor as well.

From there, Peter expressed his thoughts about his parents' expectations of him. He indicated that his father tried to draw him into a pact to hide things from his mother. The counselor let that go without comment, leaving the matter without further clarification. Was it entirely Peter's father's idea? Did Peter agree or disagree or have any other reaction(s) to this? By simply asking Peter how he felt about that sort of business in his family, the counselor would have begun to get an idea of how Peter participated emotionally in the family communication system, as well as some information about his activity in it. As observers of the interview, we can already see Peter's tendency to see himself as passive in the family and acted upon, although the counselor has not yet chosen to question that point.

The counselor's next comment, indicating that a pattern of communication would take time to change, explicitly indicated what Peter's goals *should be*, when she should have been attempting to find out what Peter's goals *are*. This comment may even have seemed to suggest that Peter had to be patient and be a good boy, which again put the counselor in the position of advisor-parent instead of objective, understanding listener.

Later on, the counselor commented that Peter was proceeding in a practical manner. Here again the counselor was judging Peter's behavior rather than trying to understand it. The counselor seems to be relying on conscious content only, i.e., Peter's overt behavior, without fully appreciating or noting the extent of his underlying conflicts and ambivalence.

This deficiency in the counselor's approach becomes clear to us when the counselor quite honestly recognized that she had become excessively concerned about Peter's behavior and found herself taking on a parental role. Chapter 2 emphasized the necessity for the therapist to keep a sharp eye on his own personal reactions that might interfere with the therapy. The exercise in self-understanding on the part of the counselor is intended to permit the counselor to return to a benevolent, objective stance. In this case, the counselor, as she clearly recognized, found herself burdening Peter with her self-awareness. Quite understandably, Peter looked disappointed. In her attempt to recover and to respond to Peter's disappointment, the counselor found herself once again judging Peter by telling him that his plan sounded sensible. Again the counselor took on a judging role instead of exploring the client's response. Although Peter apparently cheered up, his comment indicated that he now saw the counselor as a judge instead of as an understanding partner in the therapeutic relationship. The counselor continued in this role by advising Peter about what to do with his father. If, instead of becoming so concerned with Peter's behavior, the counselor had thought through how Peter's concern about his parents' expectations fitted into his general structure, that is, to what extent Peter's well-being was dependent on his being seen by significant others as a "good boy," the counselor could not only have pointed out to Peter the extent to which his desire for goodness was influencing his life, but also prepared him for a similar experience in the counseling situation.

The counselor attempted to get back to Peter's inner life, and for the first time in the interview tried to offer Peter a chance to express his feelings about leaving home. With her question, the counselor recognized that Peter was in conflict about the move and had mixed feelings. Peter responded to this, first by agreeing, then by becoming silent, and then by getting somewhat anxious. At that point the counselor again burdened Peter with her own experience. Peter ostensibly brightened at having so sympathetic a listener. But as observers, we can guess that if what Peter had wanted was a sympathetic friend, he would not have come to see a counselor. That assumption is strongly supported by Peter's reluctance to make another appointment.

FIRST INTERVIEW—B

The following selection is taken from the beginning counselor's report of his first interview. In this case it is also the client's first interview.

Ms. Stewart, an attractive 24-year-old woman, was referred to me for counseling by an emergency ward following a suicide attempt. When Ms. Stewart entered the office, I asked her to have a seat. I said that we would talk today mainly about her background. I explained that I needed to know this in order to help her solve her problems. She said that she had just had a meeting with some doctors and nurses who had asked her a lot of ridiculous questions. I asked her what some of the questions were. She listed them off as "How did I feel when I took the pills?" "Why was I depressed?" "Had I felt that way before?" She did not know how to answer the questions. She did not remember how she had felt when she took the pills. I realized that Ms. Stewart was trying to tell me she wasn't ready to talk about her suicide attempt.

So I changed the subject and asked her to tell me a little about herself, where she was raised, where she went to school, etc. She related that she was born and raised in Connecticut. She has a younger sister who is 21 years old and married. Without further discussion of her family, she said she had been an excellent student in high school and had gone on to become a laboratory technician. I asked her if her parents approved. She said it didn't matter much to them but she supposed that they were glad she had a career. I asked her what she had done after she graduated from school. She had worked at a local hospital and then moved to California, where she easily got a job in another hospital.

We discussed her experience as a laboratory technician at some length. I asked her why she went to California in the first place. She said that she wanted to see the country. She had never been outside of Connecticut and thought that this would be a good way to do it. I asked her if she liked it in California. She said no, not really, as it was not what she had hoped for. I asked her why. She described the jobs she was given as being below her ability. She didn't like taking orders from her supervisor, nor did she like to give orders to the aides. I said I didn't understand and asked if she could tell me more. She related that instead of working directly with the patients she had to do a lot of administrative paper pushing. This was too much responsibility and she couldn't handle it.

I asked if she had any good experiences at her work. No, she couldn't think of any. She said that, fortunately, the social life in California was pretty good. I asked her to tell me more about it. She said it was great. There were lots of parties and other social activities. She dated mainly other hospital workers. Her boyfriend, to whom she had almost been engaged, worked as a hospital administrator.

I then asked her about her social life in high school. She said that she had dated some but did not have a steady boyfriend. I asked her if she would describe her childhood. She related that she was a very friendly child until about age 8, when all of a sudden she became shy. I asked what she meant, and she explained that she stayed home after school and watched TV and ate until she got fat and ugly. I asked her how she felt about that. She said that people made fun of her and she retreated even more. Her family also joked about her and called her names. I asked how she felt about her family calling her names. She said that she did not become bothered by it at first but after a while she felt hurt.

Finally when she was around age 13 she decided to lose weight. I asked why she decided to lose weight then. She was a junior in high school and had begun to take an interest in boys and wanted to be more attractive to them. When asked if she dated much, she said no but she did date a little, but no one serious. I asked if she had many friends. She said not many. She did have one special guy that she dated in high school, but he wasn't a steady boyfriend. Recently she heard that he was killed in an automobile accident. I asked if that upset her. She said it did, especially since she had known him so well. I asked her to tell me more about her high school years—what activities she was involved in? She liked sports because she liked to win and worked very hard to do so. I asked what happened when she lost. She explained that she became quiet and usually walked away. I asked if she became hostile toward the winner. She said she didn't, she just got depressed. In fact, she's been depressed for a few years now, and that's why she took the pills.

We then switched to her current situation, and I asked her to tell me more about her taking the pills. She explained that the whole thing started when her boyfriend broke up with her and married someone else. This really upset her. However, she didn't express it by crying. Ms. Stewart said she realizes now that her problem is that she keeps things inside and lets them boil. I asked her what happened then. She decided to leave California and come to Boston where she easily obtained work at a hospital. She started dating, but after each date she'd return to her apartment and feel depressed. I asked about what. She said she pretended to have fun on dates but she really didn't care about any of the guys. I asked if she ever talked to her friends or family about her depression, and she said no, she just kept it all inside.

I asked her when she took the pills for the first time. She explained that 4 months ago she took a handful of phenobarbital pills after the man she had been dating told her he didn't want to see her anymore. Her roommate found her and took her to the emergency ward. Things went OK for a while after that until two weeks ago when she again took an overdose of sleeping pills.

Her most recent suicide attempt was explained in some detail. She had been asked to leave her job when a friend with whom she worked falsely accused her of stealing. In dismissing her, her supervisor implied that because she had had previous psychological problems it would be better if she left work. Again I asked Ms. Stewart if she had talked to anyone about this, and again she said no, she just kept it all inside. She returned to her apartment and again resorted to pills. Ms. Stewart said she knows there is something wrong with her. She didn't really want to die and realizes that she needs help in getting out of her depression. I asked how often she got depressed. She said quite often. She's been depressed since her boyfriend broke up with her. She puts everything into a relationship, and when things go wrong, she takes it as a personal rejection. After a silence, I told Ms. Stewart that she and I would be meeting on a regular basis to discuss her problems. I asked her what day she preferred to come in. She said she wasn't sure which day she'd be able to get a ride to the clinic. I told her I would call her in a few days to discuss an appointment time. She agreed, and we said goodbye.

Discussion

The counselor began the first interview by indicating to the client in a very specific way exactly what they were going to talk about: Ms. Stewart's background. With this instruction the counselor not only indicated a very tightly structured interview and a very controlling position, but also, and more important, he neglected to find out what was going on with Ms. Stewart and what her understanding was of this interview. In almost all situations, it is important to know what brought the client into the office at this time—from the client's point of view. It is an easy question to ask and one that clients understand.

The counselor attempted to explain this tight structure, but, in doing so, promised to "solve" Ms. Stewart's problems if the proper information was forthcoming. The client talked about a number of people who had asked ridiculous and useless questions, showing that we as counselors can rely on an intrinsic interest on the part of the client to tell us what is going on. It would have been appropriate for the counselor to ask Ms. Stewart if she felt that their own interchange thus far had made sense. Although the counselor did not pick up on that particular bit of interaction, he did recognize what Ms. Stewart was trying to say at an unconscious level. That is, he did not rely solely on her words—the conscious content—but recognized that her complaints about people indicated that she was not ready to talk about her suicide attempt.

Recognizing the blocks, the counselor sensitively changed the subject and began asking a series of open-ended questions to develop a coherent story of Ms. Stewart's life. Along the way, he did stumble a couple of times. When he asked Ms. Stewart if she liked living in California, the question really permitted only a yes or no answer. A broader question would have been "What were the things you liked and disliked in California?" The broader question permits the client to select the things more emotionally relevant at this particular time and also indicates by its very nature that people feel more than one way about things at the same time. The counselor also asked questions beginning with "Why," which, as discussed earlier, are to be avoided.

A moment or so later, however, when Ms. Stewart was indicating how difficult it was for her to be in either a dominant or submissive position, the counselor asked for more information which gave the client a chance to elaborate. Unfortunately, the counselor next asked if the client had had good experiences at work, thus falling back into the trap of asking a question requiring only a yes or no answer. It is important to note that the client's answer to these questions was always no. This is understandable in a depressed client who, as a result of her condition, sees the world very darkly indeed. Therefore, another reason to avoid yes or no questions is that the counselor knows he is likely to get a negative answer. But if his question implies that there are both active positive and active negative feelings, he is, in effect, indicating to the client that things are not always as bleak as they seem now.

Despite occasional lapses the counselor continued to get the client to say more about how she felt about her childhood and her family. Slowly the interview got into Ms. Stewart's feelings of sadness—which came out particularly around the death of a friend. While discussing the whole area of her depression, the counselor asked her if in contests she became hostile toward the winner. That might be an appropriate question for a client that the counselor knew quite well. But with a depressed client that the counselor is seeing for the first time, it is far safer to simply ask, "How did you feel about someone who beat you?" instead of leading the client toward angry feelings.

Depressed clients are hard to interview, and the counselor often has a strong desire to think of ways that might alleviate the dark mood. Again and again the counselor asked Ms. Stewart if she talked with anyone about her depression. Asked once, this question would be appropriate to elicit information about the client's interaction with friends and family. But asked repeatedly, this question implies that she should be talking with people about these depressed feelings, and further that it could be good for her if she did. While some people would consider this a reasonable suggestion, others would consider talking out their problems with friends and family impossible. As stated earlier, the counselor should not tell the client what to do. What the counselor should have done at that point was find out how Ms. Stewart felt about her depression and what her ideas were for dealing with it.

Despite these lapses, the client and counselor got along sufficiently well for Ms. Stewart to begin to tell him about her attempts at suicide. Up to this point, the material presented by the client had given little to indicate what might have led her to so serious an act as attempted suicide. After talking about the specific situations that had led to her suicide attempts, Ms. Stewart began to make some comments indicating that she felt there was something wrong with her and that she put an excessive value on certain relationships. At this time the counselor should not have implied that he had a solution, such as meeting regularly to discuss the client's problems. He should instead have conveyed to the client that he understood her feelings. A question such as "Is that how you think of yourself?" could have begun to elicit the kind of information that would give the counselor a chance to show that he understood. The counselor could point out that the overevaluation of certain relationships is an indication of the client's underevaluation of herself.

At the end of the interview, the counselor should have asked the client how she felt about their meeting before arranging the next appointment. However, many beginning counselors have considerable trouble ending their first interview. They find it easier to just tell the client the time and date of the next meeting and to ignore the importance of asking the client how he feels about meeting, what he thinks might be accomplished, and what ideas he has on how to go about it. It is always more difficult to deal with ambiguity and ambivalence and the initial questions of the client, such as "What good will talking do?" "How long will it go on?" "What am I supposed to do?" However, when these and similar questions are worked through (see the section on working through in Chap. 3), the client and the counselor are far more likely to mutually agree to meet and work together.

9
TERMINATION

The stage for termination is set during the initial interview, when the working agreement and the goals for treatment are agreed upon. The clarity with which the client and the counselor have developed the treatment objectives influences the decision and the timing of termination.

EMOTIONS SURROUNDING TERMINATION

Termination evokes a variety of emotions on the part of both the client and the counselor. Terminating a relationship revives feelings regarding previous separations and losses. These vary from anger, rejection, abandonment, sadness, and guilt to relief, pleasure, and a sense of independence, and a sense of accomplishment.

When the client has shown a great deal of response and improvement, and working with him has been rewarding for the counselor, the counselor sometimes finds it difficult to terminate. This may result in the counselor's holding on to the client longer than is necessary. Conversely, a counselor may terminate early when he thinks that the treatment is not going well or that he has little rapport with the client. Discussion of his feelings with his supervisor may make it possible for the counselor to deal with his own conflicts. He will then be less likely to terminate early or to interfere with the client's efforts to terminate when the goals have been reached.

Clients may become defensive and deny that termination is a significant experience or that they have any feelings connected with it. When this occurs, the counselor encourages the expression of feelings by asking such questions as "What thoughts are you having about terminating?" "What has the experience meant to you?" "What ways do you think you can use what you have learned in the future?" Regardless of whether the treatment was brief or long-term, the client has usually invested a good deal of energy and effort in it. He is interested and involved in what has been transpiring, and although he may deny it, he is reluctant to give up this special investment in looking at himself. In longer-term counseling, feelings around termination are usually more intense and require about 4 to 6 weeks of discussion for resolution.

TERMINATION AFTER BRIEF TREATMENT

Some clients are seen for crisis intervention or for brief treatment for a period of 1 to 3 months. Usually brief treatment is handled on a time-limited basis. Thus, both counselor and client are aware of the length of treatment and are prepared for the time of separation from the outset. Sometimes this leads to termination being the main issue of treatment. More often only parts of the last few sessions are devoted to issues about termination, with the major focus on future plans and ways the client has of coping with his situation.

RESISTANCE TO TERMINATION

As part of the process of termination, clients often react with some form of regression, such as a recurrence of symptoms. Clients, in their unconscious efforts to prolong the relationship, may bring up new problems that need to be worked on or old problems that they refrained from bringing up in the past. When clients show regressive behavior or present new problems, the counselor points this out as a resistance to terminating. If termination is to proceed, it is not a good idea for the counselor to make an effort to work on these new problems. When termination has been agreed upon by both parties, the best procedure is to stop counseling despite any exacerbations of symptoms. However, it is reasonable to make a follow-up appointment for two or three months later. Thus, if the recently increased conflicts have not settled down, the counselor is in a position to arrange a consultation with another counselor or, in rare instances, to resume the counseling.

TERMINATION BY MUTUAL AGREEMENT

Ideally, termination occurs upon mutual agreement when the client and counselor feel that much has been done and that what the client wants to continue to understand may be done as well or better on his own. The idea for terminating may be initiated by either the client or the counselor. The counselor usually responds to cues from the client that he understands his problems better and feels they are manageable. Under these circumstances it is possible to review with the client what has been accomplished, what is still left to do, and what his expectations of the future are.

TERMINATION PROVOKED BY A DISAGREEMENT

Termination sometimes occurs when there is a disagreement between the client and counselor and may be initiated by either party. A client may discontinue treatment because he is dissatisfied or feels hopeless. When a client is dissatisfied the counselor can suggest a consultation and the possibility of a referral. When a client denies his illness by a "flight into health," the counselor may have no choice but to agree to terminate and encourage the client to return at a future date if he so wishes.

CLINICAL REASONS FOR TERMINATION

A counselor may initiate termination because of clinical reasons when he feels the counseling is not going well. In these instances the counselor may request a consultation with a senior or more experienced colleague for advice regarding the counseling. In such situations the counselor explains to the client his reasons for the consultation in order to obtain the client's permission and cooperation as well as to lessen the client's feeling of rejection, failure, or worthlessness.

After the client's permission is obtained, the counselor follows the agency procedures regarding such requests. If there are no prescribed channels, the counselor reviews the case with his supervisor or another experienced colleague for further guidance regarding the handling of the case.

TERMINATION DUE TO OUTSIDE FACTORS

Outside factors such as relocation can force termination. When the counselor initiates termination because of relocation or other personal reasons, the client is likely to experience feelings of abandonment, anger, and negativism. This sometimes arouses guilt in the counselor for leaving the client in such a vulnerable position. If the client accepts a transfer to another counselor, the issue of transfer can become a useful part of the treatment.

A POSITIVE VIEW OF TERMINATION

Because the process of termination is rarely entirely smooth, a beginner can become very discouraged when trying to work it out with his client. Usually beginners as well as clients have invested a good deal of energy and time, which often results in the client's showing exceptional improvement. The period of termination, with its concomitant side effects for both the client and the counselor, is likely to be emotionally trying. However, there are some things to keep in mind that may help to ease the situation. Even though the client and the counselor stop working together, in many instances the client has a new capacity for perceiving the world and new ways of thinking and functioning autonomously. It may be hoped and often assumed that these new capacities are integrated into the individual, and he will take them with him wherever he goes regardless of whether he ever sees the counselor again. From time to time the client may make contact with his counselor and so, too, the counselor with the client. Such contacts may be made over the telephone, in person, or by letters. But whether the counselor and the client actually communicate or not, the quality of the therapeutic relationship lasts beyond the termination as they both draw from what they have learned from the counseling and from each other.

10
GETTING THE MOST OUT
OF SUPERVISION

In most agencies, provision is made for supervision of beginning counselors. If a beginner finds that this is not provided, he must insist that some arrangement for supervision be made as it is unfair to both the client and the counselor if proper safeguards are not available. There are several methods of supervision, and, no matter what the method, the general principles behind supervision are accepted by most authorities.

THE FUNCTIONS OF SUPERVISION

Supervision has two basic functions: administrative and educational. The main administrative purpose is accountability for delivery of service through assuring a high degree of competence and ethics and through fiscal responsibility. The requirements for this accountability are:

1. The supervisor and counselor together evaluate the counselor's performance and, when applicable, decide about promotions and raises.
2. The counselor adheres to the agency's procedures for statistics and record keeping.

3. The counselor adheres to the agency's policies and standards for personnel.
4. The counselor participates and demonstrates interest in the ongoing business of the agency.

The educational functions of supervision are:

1. To aid the counselor in exploring and integrating a body of knowledge and theory.
2. To facilitate the development of the counselor's skills in practice.
3. To increase the counselor's understanding of the client's situation.
4. To increase the counselor's awareness of his role in and his effect on the treatment situation.

The educational function of supervision provides the counselor with the opportunity to develop his skills as a professional counselor. The extent of that development is a personal matter and is an essential part of the counselor's sense of professional integrity and pride.

In order to provide better services to the client as well as for the counselor's sense of professionalism, the counselor is advised to take an active, rather than reactive, part in the supervisory process. The counselor knows best what he needs to work on and to learn. The wise supervisor will support and encourage the self-directed beginning counselor.

CONCERNS OF THE BEGINNING COUNSELOR

An agenda formulated by the beginning counselor is an aid in preparation both for the supervisor and the counselor, or supervisee, for a thorough discussion of the concerns being raised. Most supervisees' concerns fall into three areas: (1) background knowledge and theory, (2) technical skills, and (3) attitudes that facilitate the learning experience. Therefore, the supervisory conference may be quite intellectual, focusing on the literature of the field, including theory and research findings, for the purpose of building the counselor's knowledge and understanding of a particular phenomenon. At another time, the conference may be very practical, focusing on the counselor's facility with technique, through examining what was good or troublesome about an interview.

Underlying the use of knowledge and specific techniques are the basic attitudes that the counselor has toward the client group. These attitudes may include prejudices, stereotypes, moralistic judgments, personal preferences, and idiosyncratic reactions stemming from the counselor's personal life experience. Because attitudes and feelings are not easily identified, special efforts must be made to review patterns of interaction, repetition of problem situations, and unusual or unproductive relationships with clients. While it is hard to be objective when examining one's own work, it is important to identify these personalized attitudes and feelings so that they will not interfere with the client's work. This is probably the most difficult aspect of supervision for both the beginning and seasoned practitioner. Sharing the process of the interview through written records provides a format for the joint review by counselor and supervisor.

A process recording consists of the recollections of the interchanges both verbal and nonverbal between the client and the counselor.[1 (pp 267-281)] Perfect recall of the session is not possible nor is it expected. It is important to include the main topics and how they are introduced and by whom. In other words, the emphasis centers on the subject matter and the emotions and gestures or affect accompanying the material. Of special concern is the way the discussion shifted and whether these shifts reflect the client's or the counselor's interests. The supervisee also summarizes his overall impressions of what has transpired and formulates the goals or next steps to be worked on.

Discussion of emotionally charged areas usually leads to their neutralization and lessens subjectivity and overidentification. In exploring subjects that are conflictual for the counselor, self-awareness often evolves. This process is educational rather than therapeutic. If there is an occasional situation in which the counselor's personal conflicts consistently interfere with the treatment, the supervisor either recommends that the client be transferred to another counselor or suggests that the counselor consider treatment for himself. Although self-examination may be difficult, it is a critical exercise for all clinicians in order for them to maximize their abilities and talents and to minimize their limitations.

Because the beginner is usually inhibited by acute self-consciousness, minute scrutiny of the counselor's performance will not be as productive as focusing on the client's conflicts and noting the counselor's spontaneous responses to them.

Bertha Reynolds suggests that once a beginner has acted in behalf of a client, the paralyzing effects of self-consciousness and anxiety are diminished.[2](pp 75-85) This is comparable to the client taking a first step in his own behalf in a beginning interview.

USING SUPERVISION

The following examples demonstrate the use of supervision to benefit both the client and the counselor.

Paul, age 16, wanted to move to a foster home as he felt his parents did not understand him and he could no longer live at home. Paul felt alienated and unable to communicate. His main complaint centered on his relationship with his mother, whom he felt was too strict and overbearing. On the surface, it seemed that Paul's mother was the cause of all his problems. However, by listening carefully to Paul's unconscious as well as his conscious associations, the counselor became aware of the possibility of an underlying sexual conflict between Paul and his mother, which suggested that Paul had a painful, ambivalent attachment to his mother and that his wish to move out was an attempt to break away from his inner involvement. Before acting on the request for a foster home, the counselor brought this case to his supervisor. Together they reviewed this complex attachment and agreed that the counselor should explore the mother-son relationship further but that he should not confront Paul with the sexual aspect of it. The supervisor indicated that a more viable parent-child relationship might be worked out if the counselor suggested to Paul that they think through together what was going on instead of Paul acting on his impulse. The counselor agreed that if the client could look at the problems he was experiencing, he might not feel it necessary to leave home.

Phyllis, age 15, wanted to obtain birth control pills. The counselor was reluctant to make a referral because she disapproved of Phyllis's sexual activity. In reviewing the case with her supervisor, the counselor realized that her own subjective response had influenced her refusal to meet the client's request. In discussing the implications of her attitudes with the supervisor, the counselor was able to gain a more neutral attitude and to modify her approach with the client.

PROBLEMS WITH SUPERVISION

It is important that the supervisor and supervisee mutually respect each other. Subtle interferences may develop when a supervisee gets overconcerned that he will offend a supervisor personally because he has different philosophical, political, or generational beliefs. These feelings need to be discussed so that they may be worked out. On rare occasions when these feelings cannot be discussed and worked out by the two parties involved, another person in the agency hierarchy may be asked to consult about this interference with training.

Although supervisors are selected for their experience and skills in practice, they are not infallible. A competent supervisor shows what reasonable progress is and points out and helps the supervisee deal with unrealistic expectations. The supervisor's administrative and evaluative responsibility guarantees him considerable authority over the counselor. Unless the supervisor recognizes this reality in the relationship and makes clear that his focus is on education and not on power, the supervisee may feel excessive pressure to conform to the supervisor's wishes. Obviously, this would interfere with the teaching and learning process.

The counselor's personal feelings may cause a problem with supervision. For example, he may have discovered that his own reactions and attitudes are getting in the way of working with the client and that he may need treatment or a psychiatric consultation. He may ask the supervisor for guidance in obtaining treatment, but he should not involve the supervisor in the details of his problem as this would set up a quasi-therapeutic relationship that could only interfere with supervision. It is the supervisor's responsibility to prevent this from happening if the supervisee does try to involve him in a personal problem. The supervisor's refusal to become involved is not a rejection of the supervisee or a lack of compassion; it is simply in the supervisee's best interest that he seek help from someone other than his supervisor.

There may be times when there is no particular problem with the supervisory relationship, but the counselor desires more stimulation than individual supervision provides. He may try to develop group supervision and reach out to his peers and others to set up regular meetings to discuss matters of practice in which they share mutual concerns. He can also engage in self-supervision through a program of reading. He can assess his own degree of knowledge and skills by making up a self-assessment form. This would consist of a list of the tasks he must perform in carrying out his job and determining his degree of skill and knowledge for each of these tasks. This provides a profile for deciding the areas in which he wishes to improve.

There may be other times when a counselor is perfectly satisfied with his supervision but concerned that the agency is not serving clients as adequately as it should. His questions can be brought to supervision but also may be raised in group supervision and in staff meetings. If the counselor appears to be griping, he will have little impact. If, however, he collects data and prepares his case well and indicates a willingness to work on the problem with others, he will usually find the administration and the rest of the staff receptive. An attitude of broad concern, beyond the immediate case, is a hallmark of a real professional.

TYPES OF SUPERVISION

The various methods and modalities for supervision depend on the specific arrangements, facilities, and purposes of each agency. Often the counselor can have a role in suggesting the type of supervision needed.

Individual Supervision

The counselor meets with the supervisor individually and reviews his cases through use of records. This is the most frequent technique. A close working relationship develops in which the participants learn how each one works and how they work together. Within this framework, they focus on understanding the client's personality, the dynamic mechanisms by which conflicts are managed, and the various technical therapeutic possibilities for that particular situation.

While audio and visual tapes may be used, usually they are not readily available to the beginner.

Direct Observation

The beginning counselor sits in or observes, through a one-way mirror, an interview being conducted by the supervisor.

Through this method the supervisor acts as a model counselor. After the session is completed, a discussion follows regarding the themes, the client's reactions, the supervisor's and the beginning counselor's techniques, including both useful maneuvers and errors.

Role Playing

The counselor takes on simulated roles to better understand the interview process or the client's feelings. For example, one counselor could act the part of a 21-year-old client who is without funds and has gone to the agency to obtain financial assistance. Another counselor could act the part of the assigned intake worker whose task is to explore eligibility. The interview situation is played out, and each counselor has the opportunity to experience what it is like to be a client in a crisis or a counselor assessing a need.

Dyadic Interviewing

Two counselors are asked to enact an initial situation in which the interviewer's responsibility is to learn as much as he can about his colleague within a specified time limit. This reveals to the counselor the various tools needed to get acquainted with and learn about another person. The interviewee is confronted with the difficulties and resistances of sharing information about himself and in the process becomes aware of the interviewer's techniques.

Peer Supervision

Counselors get together either formally or informally to discuss and share common experiences. This affords a great deal of mutual support and morale building. Discussions with peers about which techniques have worked and which ones have failed lead to more openness and less concern about criticism by those higher in the organizational structure.

Group Supervision

In one form of group supervision, a supervisor discusses the common problems of the counselors didactically. In the second form the group itself plays a dynamic part in the learning. The group experience increases the individual counselors' awareness of ways of interacting as well as providing a laboratory for demonstration of group process.

Consultation

When there is a special problem that has been unresolved in the client's treatment, an expert is selected to review and give advice on the case. Consultants can be of assistance in determining the extent of pathology, uncovering the issues that keep the client from improving, or in recommending different treatment techniques.

Seminars and Workshops

Many agencies provide formal learning experiences as part of staff development programs. Seminars are designed for sharing knowledge; workshops are for work on a particular problem. These and other forms of group learning opportunities are usually based on the participant's needs.

SUPERVISION AND SELF-DEVELOPMENT

No matter what the chosen method of supervision, the beginner who invests in it as a means of improving the way he works with a client will find it an important and enriching experience. Through it, he will have the opportunity to discuss his practice with another professional and thereby avoid misunderstandings and mistakes that, when undetected, are easily reinforced by repetition. Reviewing the details with a supervisor will often disclose dynamics within the case or within the counselor that otherwise are apt to be neglected or overlooked.

With increasing experience the counselor will be better able to examine his own performance. Together with the supervisor, an evaluation will be done in which reasonable standards for the counselor's work will be set. The more the counselor can pinpoint where he is in his experience, the more he can plan ahead in directing his own learning and developing his skills. Such self-direction assures that the evaluation will be an educational and enriching process for the supervisee.

Supervision is essential for the beginner. If he approaches it as an opportunity for self-development, he will maximize all means of learning from it. Eventually, as he becomes a skilled practitioner, he will have mastered the techniques of self-directed learning and will be ready for more independent practice. Just as the goal of counseling is to enable the client to function independently, so too, the long-range goal of supervision is for the counselor to function on his own.

REFERENCE

1. Ekstein R, Wallerstein RS: The Teaching and Learning of Psychotherapy. New York, Basic Books, 1959
2. Reynolds BC: Learning and Teaching in the Practice of Social Work. New York, Rinehart, 1942

INDEX